Advanced Information
and Knowledge Processing

Series Editors

Professor Lakhmi Jain
Lakhmi.jain@unisa.edu.au
Professor Xindong Wu
xwu@cems.uvm.edu

For other titles published in this series, go to
http://www.springer.com/series/4738

Maurice D. Mulvenna · Chris D. Nugent
Editors

Supporting People with Dementia Using Pervasive Health Technologies

Foreword by June Andrews

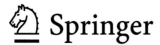 Springer

Editors
Professor Maurice D. Mulvenna
TRAIL Living Lab
School of Computing and Mathematics
Faculty of Computing and Engineering
University of Ulster
Shore Road
Newtownabbey
Northern Ireland, UK
BT37 0QB
md.mulvenna@ulster.ac.uk

Professor Chris D. Nugent
Computer Science Research Institute
School of Computing and Mathematics
Faculty of Computing and Engineering
University of Ulster
Shore Road
Newtownabbey
Northern Ireland, UK
BT37 0QB
cd.nugent@ulster.ac.uk

ISSN 1610-3947
ISBN 978-1-4471-2537-2   e-ISBN 978-1-84882-551-2
DOI 10.1007/978-1-84882-551-2
Springer London Dordrecht Heidelberg New York

British Library Cataloguing in Publication Data
A catalogue record for this book is available from the British Library

Printed on acid-free paper

Springer is part of Springer Science+Business Media (www.springer.com)

Foreword

You may have picked up this book without knowing what "pervasive computing technology is". Like me, you might think of using the pervasive technology in your life to find out. There, on the Internet, I discovered about mHealth and the use of mobile electronic devices for supporting public health and health care. I realised that I knew about all of this, all along. I just called it something else. I use my handheld electronic Sudoku to relax and my electronic diary to remember things. My hands-free car phone keeps me in touch with the family and fills in the long hours on the motorway, and lets me leave the office earlier. When I get dementia, which is a 50% possibility if I am lucky enough to reach 95 years old, I want to do as much as possible to care for myself, using technology with which I will be familiar. Even now, when I cannot find my reading glasses, why does my microwave rely on me being able to read the instructions for heating up my meal for one? Let the machine do it, please. I have got more important things to do with my life.

Care for people with dementia is, above all, about communication. The person with dementia is usually an older person, with the common sensory and physical impairments that often come with ageing, but with a reduced capacity to deal with them. Historically there has been very little information about dementia and how a person can live well with dementia. Thankfully dementia strategies internationally are making this better, but we still have a generation of health and social care workers who share a nihilistic view about the condition. Because the new information sources for carers are usually accessed after signposting from health and social care professionals, there is a delay in getting vital information and support out into systems. Now we recognise that the diagnosis of dementia is the first step towards being able to access help and support. Those charged with making a diagnosis are being asked to do it earlier and earlier, so the demand is going to rise even faster than the rise in prevalence of the condition.

This is one reason why this book is timely and exciting. Technology offers support for a number of the challenges of dementia. How can I deal with my memory not being so good? How can I stay in touch with the people who love me? What is there for me to do when my old past times start to get too difficult? This book could not be published at a better time. For those who are caring for others, or caring for themselves, it is vital that we use everything which is already at our disposal to make living with dementia easier. In the future, particularly when there may be a reduction in the resource for public services, our quality of life will depend on it.

Stirling, Scotland   June Andrews

Contents

Contributors

Anna-Lena Andersson Centre for Distance-Spanning Healthcare, Luleå University of Technology; Lighthouse, Social Welfare Services City of Luleå, Luleå, Sweden, anna-lena.andersson@soc.lulea.se

Susanne Andersson Division of Medical Specialities, Norrbotten County Council, Luleå, Sweden, susanne.b.andersson@nll.se

Matthias Baumgarten TRAIL Living Lab, School of Computing and Mathematics, Faculty of Computing and Engineering, University of Ulster, Newtownabbey, Northern Ireland, m.baumgarten@ulster.ac.uk

Johan E. Bengtsson Centre for Distance-Spanning Healthcare, Luleå University of Technology, Luleå, Sweden, johan.e.bengtsson@cdt.ltu.se

Sanne Bentvelzen Department of Psychiatry, Alzheimer Center (EMGO-Institute), VU University Medical Center, Amsterdam, The Netherlands, s.bentvelzen@vumc.nl

Birgitta Bergvall-Kåreborn Centre for Distance-Spanning Healthcare, Luleå University of Technology, Sweden, birgitta.bergvall-kareborn@ltu.se

William Burns School of Computing and Mathematics, University of Ulster, Jordanstown, UK, wp.burns@ulster.ac.uk

David Craig Department of Elderly Care, School of Medicine, Belfast City Hospital/Queen's University, Belfast, Northern Ireland (UK), david.craig@qub.ac.uk

Richard Davies Computer Science Research Institute and School of Computing and Mathematics, University of Ulster, Jordanstown, UK, rj.davies@ulster.ac.uk

Mark Donnelly Computer Science Research Institute and School of Computing and Mathematics, University of Ulster, Jordanstown, UK, mp.donnelly@ulster.ac.uk

Rose-Marie Dröes Academic Department of Psychiatry, Regional Institute for Mental Health Services GGZ-Buitenamstel Geestgronden/EMGO-Institute, VU University Medical Center, Amsterdam, The Netherlands, rm.droes@vumc.nl

Angele Giuliano AcrossLimits Technologies LTD, Gateway Centre, HMR10 Hamrun, Malta, angele@acrosslimits.com

Marike Hettinga Novay, Enschede, The Netherlands, marike.hettinga@novay.nl

Halgeir Holthe University Hospital of North Norway/Norwegian Centre for Telemedicine (NST), Tromsø, Norway, halgeirh@hholthe.no

Jeffrey Kaye Departments of Neurology and Biomedical Engineering, Oregon Center for Aging and Technology, Oregon Health and Science University, Portland, OR, USA, kaye@ohsu.edu

Steve Lauriks Academic Department of Psychiatry, Regional Institute for Mental Health Services GGZ-Buitenamstel Geestgronden/EMGO-Institute, VU University Medical Center, Amsterdam, The Netherlands, s.lauriks@gmail.com

Ricardo Castellot Lou Telefonica I+D, Parque Tecnológico Walqa – Ed. 1, 22197 Cuarte (Huesca), Spain, rcl@tid.es

Suzanne Martin TRAIL Living Lab, School of Health Sciences, Faculty of Life and Health Sciences, University of Ulster, Jordanstown, Northern Ireland, s.martin@ulster.ac.uk

Franka Meiland Department of Psychiatry, Alzheimer Center (EMGO-Institute), VU University Medical Centre/Regional Institute for Mental Health Services GGZ-in Geest, Amsterdam, The Netherlands, fj.meiland@vumc.nl

Ferial Moelaert Telematica Institute, The Netherlands, ferial.moelaert@novay.nl

Maurice D. Mulvenna TRAIL Living Lab, School of Computing and Mathematics, Faculty of Computing and Engineering, University of Ulster, Jordanstown, UK, md.mulvenna@ulster.ac.uk

Chris D. Nugent School of Computing and Mathematics and Computer Science Research Institute, University of Ulster, Jordanstown, UK, cd.nugent@ulster.ac.uk

Peter Passmore Department of Elderly Care, School of Medicine, Belfast City Hospital/Queen's University, Belfast, Northern Ireland (UK), p.passmore@qub.ac.uk

Annika Reinersmann Academic Department of Psychiatry, Regional Institute for Mental Health Services GGZ-Buitenamstel Geestgronden/EMGO-Institute, VU University Medical Center, Amsterdam, The Netherlands, annika.reinersmann@googlemail.com

Stefan Sävenstedt Centre for Distance-Spanning Healthcare, Luleå University of Technology, Luleå, Sweden, stefan.savenstedt@ltu.se

Sharon Stephens School of Computing and Mathematics, University of Ulster, Jordanstown, UK, sstephens041@antrimgrammar.antrim.ni.sch.uk

Henriëtte Geralde van der Roest Academic Department of Psychiatry, Regional Institute for Mental Health Services GGZ-Buitenamstel Geestgronden/EMGO-Institute, VU University Medical Center, Amsterdam, The Netherlands, hg.vanderroest@vumc.nl

Jonathan Wallace TRAIL Living Lab, School of Computing and Mathematics, Faculty of Computing and Engineering, University of Ulster, Jordanstown, UK, jg.wallace@ulster.ac.uk

Part I
Background

Chapter 1
Supporting People with Dementia Using Pervasive Healthcare Technologies

Maurice D. Mulvenna, Chris D. Nugent, Ferial Moelaert, David Craig, Rose-Marie Dröes, and Johan E. Bengtsson

Abstract In this chapter, an introduction is provided into pervasive healthcare technology, specifically as the use of information and communications technology in support of European policies, primarily inclusion. The focus of the chapter, and indeed the book, is on how such technologies can support people suffering from debilitating diseases including Alzheimer's. The work describes a research project called COGKNOW, comprising a multidisciplinary research consortium of scientists from across Europe, and relates some of the early achievements of the group from some very different perspectives, including technical, clinical, ethical, and of course how the needs of people with dementia and their carers can be harnessed in the development process to produce pervasive healthcare technology and services that are valued by all the stakeholders in the process.

1.1 Introduction

In Europe by 2050, it is estimated that one-third of Europe's population will be over 60. The number of "oldest old" aged 80+ is expected to grow by 180% (Eurostat 2002). For example, in 1951, there were 300 people aged 100 and over in the UK. By the year 2031, it is estimated that this figure could boom to 36,000 (BBC 2007). Life expectancy has been rising on average by 2.5 years per decade in Europe. There are 5.5 million cases of Alzheimer's disease in Europe and more new cases per year.

Technology has the potential to improve and extend the quality of life of older people and people with disabilities by helping them to lead fuller and more independent lives. It can also improve the efficiency and effectiveness of services provided to older people and people with disabilities and so help to constrain the cost and

M.D. Mulvenna (✉)
TRAIL Living Lab, School of Computing and Mathematics, Faculty of Computing and Engineering, University of Ulster, Jordanstown, UK
e-mail: md.mulvenna@ulster.ac.uk

M.D. Mulvenna, C.D. Nugent (eds.), *Supporting People with Dementia Using Pervasive Health Technologies*, Advanced Information and Knowledge Processing, DOI 10.1007/978-1-84882-551-2_1, © Springer-Verlag London Limited 2010

improve the quality of care. Such technology can also extend their economically active life. Technology has significant potential for curbing the ever-increasing costs of caring for the elderly and the disabled.

The technical concept in COGKNOW is to develop a portable, remotely configurable mobile device and service which does not require complicated instructions or manipulations on the part of the elderly citizen, but which can aid the citizen to navigate through their day, unobtrusively offering information and reassurance, while allowing the citizen to structure their timetable and to retain greater control over their daily life activities. The consequences for greater autonomy and the empowerment to control one's own life into old age are considerable.

The core scientific and technological objective of COGKNOW is to achieve a breakthrough in the development of a successful, user-validated cognitive prosthetic device with associated services for people with mild dementia. This entails cognitive reinforcement in the four main areas of helping people to remember, helping to maintain social contact, helping with performing daily life and recreational activities, and providing enhanced feelings of safety (Meiland et al. 2007). In the COGKNOW project, we have sought to address this core objective by focusing on scientific and technological objectives for the device, including remotely configurable reminding functionality, communication and interaction functionality, supportive technology for performing Activities of Daily Living (ADLs), and anomaly detection and emergency contact.

1.2 Why Select Mild Dementia?

The choice of application area (elderly people with mild dementia) was chosen in response to the knowledge of the growing presence of this condition in an increasingly ageing population; of the Europe-wide presence of this condition and of the "demographic time-bomb" which threatens in the near future if measures are not taken to support elderly people with mild dementia to increase their autonomy and self-help; of the common need being perceived across Europe to find remedies to ameliorate the effects of dementia; and of the potential in reduction of healthcare costs by allowing the citizen to remain in their own home environment unassisted by carers for longer than would currently be the case.

Dementia is a progressive, disabling, chronic disease affecting 5% of all persons above 65 and over 40% of people over 90 years (Fratiglioni et al. 2000; Launer and Hofman 2000). The term dementia refers to a combination of symptoms involving impairments of memory, speech, thought, perception, and reasoning. Early impairments in performing complex tasks lead to an inability to perform even the most basic functional activities such as washing and eating. Often there are changes in personality, behaviour, and psychological functioning, such as depressive symptoms, apathy, and aggression. These neuropsychiatric symptoms appear to afflict the overwhelming majority of sufferers and are reported to be particularly potent precipitants of institutionalisation (Craig et al. 2005; Mirakhur et al. 2004).

The most prevalent type of dementia in the elderly is Alzheimer's disease (AD). Two-thirds of older people and one-third of younger patients (50–65 years old) with dementia have Alzheimer's disease. We propose to develop COGKNOW in a cohort of AD patients with mild impairments in cognition and function. Alzheimer's disease sufferers represent by far the most common cause of dementia throughout Europe and display a clinical course that is typically only slowly progressive. This allows the user to enjoy the eventual benefits of COGKNOW over a longer time frame (until that point is reached when severe disability intervenes) and also permits better standardisation during COGKNOW field trials where a rapidly fluctuating clinical course might impede the assessment of user need and system efficacy.

There exist relatively few studies in which persons with dementia were surveyed and allowed to describe their own specific unmet needs. Aside from physical problems (such as loss of eyesight and hearing and incontinence) the most frequently identified unmet needs are in the areas of information (on condition, treatment, care and support possibilities, appointments with care services, etc.), memory problems, and communication and psychological distress (anxiety) (Walters et al. 2000; Beattie et al. 2002, 2004; van der Roest et al. 2005). A report examining quality of life issues of dementia sufferers has recently identified seven key domains (Dröes et al. 2005): physical and mental health, social contact with family and friends, being useful to others, enjoyment of activities, self-esteem (being respected by others), and self-determination and freedom.

A different personal perspective and lack of insight into their predicament cause patients to report less needs, and in some cases different needs, than their carers (Hancock et al. 2003; van der Roest et al. 2005). In one study the needs identified by the informal carers were associated with their own mental health (Hancock et al. 2003), suggesting that the greater need of the carers could also be related with the mental health problems of the carers themselves. Unmet needs mentioned by both patients and carers include

- Memory problems of the person with dementia,
- Communication,
- (Enough) meaningful activities during day time,
- (Feelings of) safety, and
- Information (on the disease, prognosis, care policy, possible care and support services, appointments).

If we analyse these needs as described above from various studies, we can see the importance of various strands of the person's life, including feeling of autonomy, that needs reinforcement of orientation in space and in time, of topographic memory and of (auto-) biographical memory, and the ability for the person to maintain contact with their social environment and improve their relationship with it and their peers. This involves not only reinforcement of identity, episodic memory, and assisting the fight against apathy, but also facilitation of all aspects of communication and motivating people to express their opinions and thoughts and wishes and fears and reinforce their feelings of social belongingness and of references that ground people temporally.

1.3 The European Policy Landscape

In Europe, policy that supports people with disabilities, ageing people, and other groupings of people that can potentially suffer from physical, digital, or social exclusion is termed "inclusion" policy. The following sections of this chapter outline the strands of this policy as they impact on "inclusion" research.

1.3.1 Demographic Ageing

Europe is an ageing continent. Of the 458 million people in Europe almost one-sixth are aged over 65, which is 76 million (European Commission 2005). It is estimated that this proportion will have risen in some Western European countries up to one in four people in 2025 (US Census 2000), with the largest increase in the oldest (80+) age group, where disability is most prevalent (Lamura 2003): The number of people aged over 80 will rise from 18.8 million today to 34.7 million in 2030, due to the ageing baby-boomer generation and a significant increase in life expectancy resulting from improved conditions of life and improved medical practice (European Commission 2005). With the increasing number of elderly the number of disabled people will also increase, which amounts to a demographic "time bomb".

These demographic changes mean that the countries of Europe can expect a massive rise in the number of older people and a corresponding increase in the number of dementia sufferers. If one considers the associated costs of community-based caring strategies and the emotional and economic burdens associated with institutionalisation, it is clear that these unfortunate individuals must be considered in the context of both national and European healthcare strategies, as well as social and economic policies.

Based on the prevalence rates of EURODEM (Hofman et al. 1991) and population statistics from Eurostat, Alzheimer Europe has estimated the number of people with dementia in the age of 30 and older in Europe as 5,709,348 (Alzheimer Europe 2005). Among the elderly population in Europe about 5% suffer from dementia (3.8 million people). This percentage is based solely on diagnosed cases. This is likely to lead to an underestimation, because many people with dementia never receive a diagnosis and it excludes those in the early stages of dementia who have not been diagnosed (Alzheimer Europe 2005). In COGKNOW, the focus has been on the real needs and wants of people with mild dementia, that is, at least half of those suffering from dementia in the elderly population. Approximately 1.9 million elderly people in Europe experience mild dementia. This is the potentially excluded section of Europe's population that the project is seeking to assist. This figure is expected to double in the coming four decades (Health Council 2002; European Commission

2005). Thus, the COGKNOW project and equivalent research have the potential for a fundamental and sustainable impact on the development of future applications and services to support ageing people with dementia and improve their quality of life.

1.3.2 The Care Burden

Due to the growing number of ageing people, there are, and will be, long waiting lists for sheltered housing projects, homes for the elderly, nursing homes, and other care facilities. The majority of people with dementia will have to "survive" in their own homes. Furthermore, most elderly people wish to stay at home as long as possible. This on the one hand releases the pressure on the nursing homes, yet generates great pressure on informal carer(s), such as spouses, children, other family members and friends, also because of the increasing shortage of professional carers. Taking care of a person with dementia is recognised as a burdensome task (European Commission 2005). Many informal carers experience negative physical, psychological, and social consequences that besides the behavioural problems of the person with dementia are important determinants of nursing home admission of the person with dementia (Teri 1997; Braekhus et al. 1998; Aalten 2004).

Research projects such as COGKNOW can potentially help to address these societal problems by investigating how technology can be used to improve the autonomy and the quality of life of elderly people, so that people with dementia can stay longer in their own homes with a better quality of life. It is to be expected that supportive measures that increase the autonomy and quality of life of the persons with dementia will not only help the patient but will also relieve the burden for the carer.

1.3.3 European Policy Areas

European policy makers face significant challenges as they strive to retain clarity and cohesiveness across the broad policy domains of *inclusion* policy and the *information* society policy.

These two policies are interweaved in parts of the major initiative "i2010: European Information Society 2010", promoting an inclusive European information society. To close the gap between the information society "haves and have-nots", in 2007 the Commission proposed a "quality of life" Information and Communication Technology (ICT) flagship initiative on technologies for an ageing society. In 2008, the Commission also proposed actions to overcome the geographic and social "digital divide", culminating in a European Initiative on e-Inclusion.

The call for proposals to which COGKNOW and other related ICT for Inclusion projects responded articulated the challenge "to develop next-generation assistive systems that empower persons with (in particular cognitive) disabilities and ageing citizens to play a full role in society, to increase their autonomy and to realize their potential".

In Europe, therefore, the European Commission is identifying areas where research can help to devise new breakthroughs using ICT to address policy challenges strategically.

1.4 Pervasive Healthcare Technology and Services

Previous research in cognitive prosthetics has delivered devices and services which have had mixed or little success when applied to actual living conditions among ageing people with dementia (Lauriks et al. 2007). However, they have proven useful in highlighting where gaps in service and autonomy may be filled. The COGKNOW project outlined in subsequent chapters is focused on addressing these gaps and on delivering pervasive healthcare services and technology that makes a difference in actual living conditions.

The analysis of the state of the art of ICT solutions by the COGKNOW consortium for dementia sufferers showed that various types of services and several products are available for all the most frequently mentioned unmet needs. In the current market there are relatively simple products such as automatic pill dispensers or telephones with the photos of the persons frequently called, which contribute to the support for memory and social contacts, to more complex and complete tracking devices, using Global Positioning Systems (GPS), that also assist in locating people with dementia when they happen to "wander". The beneficial effects of computer systems have been observed on orientation, feelings of anxiety, and independency in patients suffering from Alzheimer's disease. Besides this, implementing monitoring technologies and detection devices or alarm systems inside and outside the home of elderly persons is potentially useful to enhance (perceived) safety and security of the person suffering from dementia as well as carers.

New technologies have also a remarkable role in assistive cares. Internet-based applications designed to provide carers with clinical, decision-making, and emotional support have been evaluated in field trials and the initial results have shown the system to be beneficial both to carers and to people with dementia (Lauriks et al. 2007). Nonetheless, despite all these pervasive healthcare services, products and technologies available to enhance and improve Alzheimer patients' quality of life, there is no system in the current market capable of offering help and solutions that cover the four main need areas previously mentioned.

This was the core rationale for the project. COGKNOW offers the potential to be a valuable approach, which implements a wide range of services that not only will help people with dementia to face up to their main needs, but also makes it possible that they can lead a normal life, included in society. The European Commission stated, "We have to apply technology to the task of genuinely empowering citizens to play a full role in society." This was our goal in COGKNOW.

The following sections outline the main areas covered by the book, namely, Sections 1.5, 1.6, 1.7, and 1.8. In each of these sections, the constituent chapters are summarised and placed in context.

1.5 Background to the Research

In this section, there are four chapters, covering medical aspects of dementia, the state of the art in electronic assistive technologies for people with dementia, a detailed chapter reviewing ICT-based services for identified unmet needs in people with dementia, and a chapter describing the issues relating to privacy, ethics, and security when designing solutions for people with dementia.

In Chapter 2, a short introduction to key aspects of this disease and its various forms is provided. The chapter begins be defining the disease and providing a historical background before describing the extent of the disease. The health economic impact of dementia is presented, together with an outline of the sub-types of dementia before the relationship between the disease and age is discussed. The risk factors associated with dementia are enumerated, and the important issue of the impact of the burden of the illness for carers and person with dementia is discussed before management aspects for the disease are presented.

In Chapter 3, the case is made of the effectiveness of pervasive healthcare technology and services in catering for the main needs of people with dementia. However, despite advances in information and communication technologies and growing sales, industry has been slow to standardise these technologies and to implement them. Because of this, in last years in Europe, there have been a large number of initiatives, both public and private, which seek to improve the situation of those persons who suffer from dementia. These initiatives and technologies are the focus of this chapter.

In Chapter 4, the authors present a systematic review of the needs of people with dementia and their carers that may be addressed by pervasive healthcare technologies and services. This chapter, then, provides an insight into the state of the art in ICT solutions that could contribute to meet the most frequently mentioned unmet needs by people with dementia and their informal carers. These needs can be summarised as the need for general and personalised information; the need for support with regard to symptoms of dementia; the need for social contact and company; and the need for health monitoring and perceived safety. The findings outlined in this chapter conclude that informational websites offer helpful information for carers but seem less attuned to the person with dementia and do not offer personalised information. The chapter also describes how ICT solutions aimed at compensating for disabilities, such as memory problems and daily activities, demonstrate that people with mild to moderate dementia are capable of handling simple electronic equipment and can benefit from it in terms of more confidence and enhanced positive affect. Finally, the chapter describes how instrumental ICT support for coping with behavioural and psychological changes in dementia is relatively disregarded as yet, while support for social contact can be effectively realised through, for example, simplified (mobile) phones or videophones or (entertainment) robots. The chapter concludes by recommending that future studies also focus on the integration of the current techniques and solutions.

In Chapter 5, pervasive healthcare technology options relating to the users are discussed before examination of the ethics, privacy, and security issues are described in detail in the context of provision of technology to assist people with dementia. New and emerging technologies provide the opportunity to develop innovative sustainable service models, capable of supporting adults with dementia at home. The findings of the chapter relate that ethical issues abound in all aspects of interventions to support adults with dementia. The chapter relates that the service context for pervasive healthcare technologies is often complex, involving a variety of stakeholders and a range of interested agencies. Against this backdrop, it is critical that due consideration is given to the potential ethical ramifications at an individual, organisational, and societal level.

1.6 The Role of the User in the Design Process

In this section, there are three chapters, examining first the identification of the needs of users in the participative design process that drives the research, how to manage the transition from the resultant user information on needs to functional requirements and subsequent technical specifications used by the system designers and finally recounting the lessons learned from field trials about which dementia-related and other factors need to be taken into account in the development process.

In Chapter 6, the process of identification of the needs of people with dementia (and their carers) is described. The design process consisted of iterative cycles at three test sites across Europe, with active participation by people with dementia and their carers in the developmental process. Based on their priorities of needs and solutions, on their disabilities and after discussion between the development team, a top four list of ICT solutions was made which served as the basis for development. These areas are in the area of remembering – day and time indication and reminding service, in the area of communication – picture dialling function, in the area of daily activities – media playback and radio function, and finally, a warning device for an open front door and an emergency help contact to enhance feelings of safety.

In Chapter 7, the management of the process that bridges the large gap between user studies and the design of the system is described. This process consists of two smaller steps: the transition from user requirements to functional requirements and from the latter to the technical specification.

Chapter 8 focuses on how issues which affect people with dementia, such as failure of prospective memory, can be taken into account as the pervasive healthcare technologies and services from COGKNOW are developed. The main dementia-related disabilities that emerged from the users and that proved relevant for the development of an assistive technological device were memory and orientation problems; poor understanding of verbal instruction; difficulty with instrumental daily activities; and recognising/understanding the meaning of pictures. Relevant personal and environmental features were living alone or with a carer; the need for company and social contact; the need for support in doing things for fun; using aids like a walking cane; possessing technological appliances that could not be easily used anymore; living in a house with multiple rooms and levels; and feeling insecure when being alone. After a development period, the user-friendliness and usefulness of the device developed to assist people with dementia were assessed via field trials. Using semi-structured interviews and observations, the experiences of the people with dementia and carers with the devices were inventoried. It was concluded that though most functions were judged as user-friendly and useful, further personalisation of the device interfaces would improve the perceived user-friendliness and usefulness. This study showed that detailed information on the functioning and living environment of the users is necessary to attune technology to their needs. The group of people with dementia that participated in this work also showed that people with mild dementia are very capable of giving their opinion on the user-friendliness and usefulness of assistive technology.

1.7 Pervasive Healthcare Technology

In this section, there are three chapters describing different aspects of the technology used in the development of a solution in the project. The role of context-aware computing in support of people with dementia is described in Chapter 9, before Chapter 10 outlines the process of prototyping and development of the technical devices and services. The final chapter in this section examines research in interface design for ageing people in general and in particular for people with dementia.

In Chapter 9, an introductory tutorial on context aware computing is provided, describing the origins of the technology and its importance with respect to location-based computing, encompassing large-scale environments as well as those of a smaller scale, such as "smart homes". The potential for computing to be able to use context-awareness information to predict such things as anticipated activities of daily living and then to offer supporting interventions is described before the applicability of such technology for people with dementia is described.

In Chapter 10, the development of a cognitive prosthetic to address the unmet needs and demands of persons with dementia through the application of ICT-based services is described. The primary aim of the developed solution was to offer guidance with conducting everyday activities for persons with dementia. The chapter describes how, to encourage a user-centred design process, a three-phased development methodology was introduced to facilitate cyclical prototype development. At each phase, user input was used to guide the future development. As a prerequisite to the first phase of development, user requirements were gathered to identify a small set of functional requirements from which a number of services were identified. Following implementation of these initial services, the prototype was evaluated on a cohort of users and, through observing their experiences and recording their feedback, the design was refined and the prototype redeveloped to include a number of additional services in the second phase.

In Chapter 11, an overview of the research and literature relating to ageing people and people with dementia is provided. The chapter also discusses the differing contexts in which ageing people interact with computerised systems and their associated issues.

1.8 Evaluation and Assessment of Cognitive Prosthetics

In this section, there are three chapters, beginning with a short chapter looking at the important practical issues involved when planning for the field trials with users. The second chapter provides a detailed examination of the process of evaluation of the cognitive prosthetics developed in the research, while the final chapter in this section describes how the COGKNOW team planned and executed the process to measure the impact of cognitive prosthetics on the daily life of people with dementia and their carers.

In Chapter 12, the role of planning and timing of field trials when testing technical solutions is described. This short chapter is written from a test site leader perspective and describes the experiences of setting up the first and second field trials in the three test sites of the COGKNOW project. The chapter addresses issues in the preparatory, the actual and the post-test phase of the field trial in order to help achieve a high level of success both from a general perspective and with a special focus on people with dementia.

In Chapter 13, the evaluation of the usefulness and user-friendliness of the first COGKNOW device is described. The chapter also draws together experiences drawn from the evaluation process, together with reflections and guidance for those contemplating field studies using pervasive healthcare technologies. The experiences from the testing process have so far shown that the use of a mix method approach using semi-structured interviews, combining structured and open questions, and semi structured observation provides a comprehensive understanding of the usefulness and user-friendliness that overcomes some of the challenges.

In Chapter 14, the COGKNOW project is used as a case study example in order to explain how the impact of cognitive prosthetics on the daily lives of people with dementia and their carers can be measured. Devices have been developed with an aim to improve the quality of life and autonomy of people with dementia and to help them to remember and remind, to have social contact, to perform daily activities, and to enhance feelings of safety. For all these areas, this chapter describes the potential instruments that can be used to measure, for example, semi-structured interviews and observations, diaries and in situ measurement.

1.9 The Way Ahead

For the final chapter, the COGKNOW researchers invited a world-respected researcher, external to the consortium, to assimilate the preceding chapters in the book, and provide a glimpse into the future of pervasive healthcare technologies and services for people with dementia.

Acknowledgement The COGKNOW project is supported by the European Commission's Information Society Technologies (IST) programme under grant 034025.

References

Aalten, P. (2004) Behavioural problems in dementia: Course and risk factors. PhD Thesis, Maastricht University, Maastricht, NL.

Alzheimer Europe. (2005) Prevalence of dementia, www.alzheimer-europe.org, 2005.

BBC. (2007) Britain's ageing population, http://news.bbc.co.uk/1/hi/health/395143.stm, accessed 6 March 2008.

Beattie, A.M., Daker-White, G., Gilliard, J., Means, R. (2002) Younger people in dementia care: A review of service needs, service provision and models of good practice. Aging & Mental Health, 6(3):205–212.

Beattie, A.M., Daker-White, G., Gilliard, J., Means, R. (2004) 'How can they tell' a qualitative study of the views of younger people about their dementia and dementia care services. Health and Social Care in the Community, 12(4):359–368.

Braekhus, A., Oksengard, A.R., Engendal, K., Laake, K. (1998) Social and depressive stress suffered by spouses of patients with mild dementia. Scandinavian Journal of Primary Health Care, 16(4):242–246.

Craig, D., Mirakhur, A., Hart, D.J., McIlroy, S., Passmore, P. (2005 Jun) A cross-sectional study of neuropsychiatric symptoms in 435 patients with Alzheimer's disease. American Journal of Geriatr Psychiatry, 13(6):460–468.

Dröes, R.M., Boelens, E.J., Bos, J., Meihuizen, L., Ettema, T.P., Gerritsen, D.L., Hoogeveen, F., de Lange, J., Schölzel-Dorenbos, C. (2005) Quality of life in dementia in perspective: An explorative study of variations in opinions among people with dementia and their professional caregivers, and in literature. Dementia (The International Journal of Social Research and Practice), in press.

European Commission. (2005) Faced with demographic change, a new solidarity between the generations: Europe's changing population structure and its impact on relations between the generations, http://europa.eu.int/rapid/pressReleasesAction, March 2005.

Eurostat. (2002) Health statistics – Key data on health 2002, http://epp.eurostat.ec.europa.eu/cache/ITY_OFFPUB/KS-08-02-002/EN/KS-08-02-002-EN.PDF, accessed 6 March 2008.

Fratiglioni, L., Launer, L.J., Anderson, K. et al. (2000) Incidence of dementia and major subtypes in Europe: A collaborative study of population-based cohorts. Neurologic Diseases in the Elderly Research Group. Neurology, 54:10–15.

Hancock, G.A., Reynolds, T., Woods, B., Thornicroft, G., Orrell, M. (2003) The needs of older people with mental health problems according to the user, the carer, and the staff. International Journal of Geriatric Psychiatry, 18:803–811.

Health Council. (2002/04) Dementia: Advice of a commission of the Health Council to the Minister of Public Health, Welfare and Sports. Den Haag, The Netherlands.

Hofman, A. et al. (1991) The prevalence of dementia in Europe: A collaborative study of 1980–1990 findings. International Journal of Epidemiology, 20(3):736–748.

Lamura, G. (2003) Supporting carers of older people in Europe: A comparative report on six European countries. Health and Social Services: Partners for a Social Europe, 11th European Social Services Conference, Venice.

Launer, L.J., Hofman, A. (2000) Frequency and impact of neurologic diseases in the elderly of Europe: A collaborative study of population based cohorts. Neurology, 54:1–13.

Lauriks, S., Reinersmann, A., van der Roest, H., Meiland, F.J.M., Davies, R.J., Moelaert, F., Mulvenna, M.D., Nugent, C.D., Dröes, R.M. (2007) Review of ICT-based services for identified unmet needs in people with dementia. Ageing Research Reviews, 6(3):223–246.

Meiland, F.J.M., Reinersmann, A., Bergvall-Kareborn, B., Craig, D., Moelaert, F., Mulvenna, M.D., Nugent, C., Scully, T., Bengtsson, J., Dröes, R.-M. (2007) COGKNOW: Development of an ICT device to support people with dementia. The Journal of Information Technology in Healthcare, 5(5):324–334.

Mirakhur, A., Craig, D., Hart, D.J., McIlroy, S., Passmore, P. (2004 Nov) Behavioural and psychological syndromes in Alzheimer's disease. International Journal of Geriatric Psychiatry, 19(11):1035–1039.

Teri, L. (1997) Behavior and caregiver burden: Behavioural problems in patients with Alzheimer disease and its association with caregiver distress. Alzheimer Disease and Associated Disorders, 11(Supp 4):S35–S38.

U.S. Census. (2000) International database, http://www.census.gov/ipc/www/idbnew.html, 2000.

van der Roest, H.G., Meiland, F.J.M., Dröes, R.M.. (2005) Needs in dementia: Preliminary results of a field study among patients and (in) formal carers. Internal Report, Department of Psychiatry, VU Medical Center, Amsterdam.

Walters, K., Iliffe, S., See Tai, S., Orrell, M. (2000) Assessing needs from patient, carer and professional perspectives: The Camberwell Assessment of Need for the Elderly people in primary care. Age and Ageing, 29:505–510.

Chapter 2
Prevalence and Clinical Features of Dementia

David Craig, Franka Meiland, Peter Passmore, and Rose-Marie Dröes

Abstract Progressive intellectual deterioration is the hallmark of dementia. Decline is normally centred around memory failure initially but virtually all cognitive capabilities are susceptible. Rapid progress in the understanding of the underlying neurobiology is currently taking place. In most instances, prevention strategies remain unclear and treatment methods are based around social and personal support as pharmacological modalities produce only modest effects. Technological means of home assistance offer a potential route towards relief of suffering and minimisation of healthcare costs.

2.1 Definition and Overview

Dementia refers to a collection of symptoms in which cognitive ability is impaired. The impairment is sufficient to create difficulty in a social or occupational context. Dementia is generally irreversible with the pattern of progression dependent on subtype. The cause of most dementias is unknown and there is no cure available other than modest symptomatic treatment.

In the case of the most common dementia, Alzheimer's disease (AD), the illness typically begins with decline in short-term memory. Other cognitive domains are affected and lead to limitation in orientation in which the affected person is unable to accurately understand the current date or appreciate his or her surroundings. Attentive capabilities may deteriorate (producing poor concentration and limited power to deal with distractions). Comprehension deficits lead to loss in understanding conversation and information that is in any way complex. If visuospatial abnormalities are present then the person may be unable to properly appreciate the

D. Craig (✉)
Department of Elderly Care, School of Medicine, Belfast City Hospital/Queen's University, Belfast, Northern Ireland (UK)
e-mail: david.craig@qub.ac.uk

M.D. Mulvenna, C.D. Nugent (eds.), *Supporting People with Dementia Using Pervasive Health Technologies*, Advanced Information and Knowledge Processing, DOI 10.1007/978-1-84882-551-2_2, © Springer-Verlag London Limited 2010

world in front of them in its true graphic form – setting the table, for example, becomes problematic because shapes and patterns become difficult or impossible to interpret (agnosia). Similarly, language abnormalities can lead to inappropriate word output as well as a decline in the meaningful interpretation of the written or spoken word as presented to the sufferer (aphasia). Finally, people will experience difficulties in manipulating objects, self-care activities and instrumental activities of daily living such as using the telephone, not through any weakness or loss of precision, rather secondary to the breakdown in higher mental sequencing and purposeful thought (apraxia).

Virtually any intellectual process is vulnerable. Although not required for the diagnosis, the vast majority of people with dementia develop behavioural and/or psychological symptoms, for example, apathy, depressive or aggressive behaviour and anxiety (Craig et al. 2005). These symptoms probably result from the combination of biological or neurochemical abnormalities with psychological and social provoking factors, such as the way the person copes with the disease and the interaction with the (at times obscure) environment. While the result of the cognitive changes is functional loss and limitation in daily activities, the psychological and behavioural symptoms result primarily in changes in personality and psychosocial functioning leading to an increased risk of placement into institutional care.

2.2 Historical Background

One of the first documented references to mental decline in old age is credited to Pythagoras who in the seventh century BC described "old age" or the senium as the period when "The scene of mortal existence closes, after a great length of time, to which, very fortunately, few of the human species arrives. The system returns to the imbecility of the first epoch of the infancy" (Jameson 1811). It is argued that Hippocrates, the "Father of Medicine", while aware of the condition of cognitive decline in the elderly, did not consider it an abnormality and did not include it in his writings of mental disorders (Berchtold and Cotman 1998). The same belief was restated by others such as Plato and Aristotle. Cicero, the Roman philosopher of the second century BC, may be the first writer of the time to argue that dementia was not an inevitable consequence of old age and was preventable via "intellectual activity which gives buoyancy to the mind", a concept furthered by Galen in the second century AD who used the specific term "morosis" in his descriptions of mental illness specific to old age (Berchtold and Cotman 1998). The application of science to the study of dementia accelerated only many years later. Benedict Morel and Samuel Wilks, in the nineteenth century, respectively, referred to weight loss affecting the brain and atrophy of the brain cortex (Berchtold and Cotman 1998). It was Alois Alzheimer in 1907 who provided vivid descriptions of the pathological changes in the demented brain of a 51-year-old lady "Auguste D" in which "fibrils" and "foci" in turn dominated the inside and outside of brain cells (Alzheimer 1907). The most perceptive aspect of Alzheimer's work other than the microscopic description was the novel contrast demonstrated between this disorder and other common illness producing cognitive decline namely vascular damage and neurosyphillis. Because of the patient's age, the disorder of Alzheimer's disease (AD) became labelled until quite recently as presenile dementia. In fact the clinicopathological features are identical in older cases. Alzheimer's represents around two-thirds of all cases of dementia.

2.3 Extent of Dementia

Prevalence estimates of dementia vary considerably between countries partly due to genuine population differences but also due to methodological variations, for example, with regard to case definition during sampling. European figures suggest that after age 65, dementia prevalence roughly doubles every 5 years. Between the ages of 65 and 69 years, dementia prevalence is 0.8% of the population, rising to 28.5% at age 90 years (Lobo et al. 2000). The incidence figures, in which the number of new cases is recorded per year, demonstrate an exponential increase in incidence with age. For example, the incidence in the 65–69 age group is 2.4 per 1,000-person years, rising to 70.2 in the 90+ age group (Fratiglioni et al. 2000). These figures impact significantly in terms of population demographics: the over-65 population is anticipated to rise from 15.4% of the EU population in 1995 to 22.4% by 2025.[1]

Based on the prevalence rates of EURODEM (Hofman et al. 1991) and population statistics from Eurostat,[2] Alzheimer Europe[3] has estimated the number of people with dementia over the age of 30 in Europe at 5.7 million. Among the elderly population (over 65) in Europe, about 5% or 3.8 million people have dementia. However, this percentage is based solely on diagnosed cases. This is likely to represent an underestimation, because many people with dementia never receive a diagnosis and it excludes those in the early stages of dementia who have not been diagnosed. At least half of those suffering from dementia in the elderly population experience mild dementia (1.9 million).

2.4 Health Economic Impact

Worldwide societal costs (2005) serving the estimated 29.3 million people with dementia were approximately US $315.4 billion in direct medical and non-medical care including informal care (Wimo and Winblad 2008). European cost-of-illness

---

[1] europa.eu/rapid/pressReleasesAction.do?reference=STAT/08/119&format=HTML&aged=0& language=EN&guiLanguage=en

[2] epp.eurostat.ec.europa.eu/portal/page?_pageid=0,1136184,0_45572592&_dad=portal& _schema=PORTAL

[3] www.alzheimer-urope.org/?lm2=283744119811&sh=6FB10D101364

studies, mostly based on retrospective resource utilisation data, present figures ranging from about €6,000 to €19,000 per person annually (Jönsson and Berr 2005).
Estimates vary between countries depending on the differences in the configuration
of care provision as well as differences in measurement criteria.

The most expensive aspect of care is associated with institutionalisation into
a residential or nursing home environment. Although cost–benefit work has only
recently begun, supporting and maintaining people within their own homes via
technological or other means are likely to produce health economic savings. A similar argument applies to delaying the onset or slowing the progression of dementia.
Identifying the most cost-effective means of achieving these biological aims is also
being actively researched.

2.5 Dementia Subtypes

While most cases of dementia represent underlying AD in pure or mixed forms,
there are other less common subtypes with distinct clinical features. AD is charac-
terised by the slow progressive loss of cognitive function frequently beginning with
decline in short-term memory. Vascular dementia (VaD) accounts for around 20–
30% of cases and frequently begins with a less subtle and more abrupt onset and
stepwise pattern of decline. Here, memory loss is a less distinctive symptom than
executive dysfunction – whereby processing and sequencing of information (and
therefore task completion) is impaired. People will therefore develop a slowness
and distractibility when attempting to function during everyday activities. Dementia
associated with the clinical features of Parkinson's disease is the third most common dementia. Physical slowness and/or tremor accompany cognitive changes
again relating to executive dysfunction but characteristic changes in visuospatial processing (graphic representation of the environment in front of the person)
are also seen. Visual hallucinations (e.g. of animals) and delusions (sometimes
of a paranoid nature) are an important neuropsychiatric symptom in this form of
dementia.

2.6 Relationship Between Normal Ageing and Dementia

Dementia accompanies ageing; however, if you live long enough you are not certain
to develop the condition. Various cognitive changes occur as we age. The fundamental difference between age-related cognitive decline and dementia is the interference
with activities of daily living either in basic (e.g. washing, dressing) or instrumental
(e.g. handling money, using the telephone). In mild forms of dementia the transition can be blurred. Cognitive impairment, for instance, existing as memory loss
demonstrable on formal testing but which fails to create significant functional consequence is now referred to as mild cognitive impairment or MCI. There is much
research exploring whether MCI is a true pre-dementia state, as seems likely, and

what factors encourage the transition to full-blown dementia (Werner and Korczyn 2008).

Similarly, even before neuropsychological testing reveals objective abnormalities in cognitive performance, the state of subjective memory impairment exists where the individual notices memory difficulties and complains that they are becoming forgetful. Whether it accounts for a possible very early "at risk" population who may later go on to develop MCI and indeed dementia is unclear. The identification of valid pre-dementia phases is important given the need to explore putative preventative strategies.

2.7 Risk Factors for Dementia

The main risk factor for dementia is age, with a slight excess risk associated with female gender. Other confirmed risk factors include a family history and possession of certain genetic markers that have a biological role in lipid metabolism. Significant head injury creates extra risk. Longer time spent in education is seemingly protective and has led to the belief that "brain training", i.e. cognitive stimulation, might delay or prevent dementia. Certainly, good mental health, and increasingly physical health, is recommended as the best guess in terms of dementia prevention. Physical variables such as high blood pressure, obesity and diabetes, once thought to be linked only to the prevention of VaD, are now considered clearly relevant to the development of AD.

Once dementia is established, the prognosis may be influenced by concurrent pathologies, e.g. stroke, neurological sequelae, e.g. loss of swallow leading to the development of aspiration and chest infection, or psychiatric symptoms such as aggression or psychosis which appear to accompany a more rapidly deteriorating disease course. External factors such as the extent of family support and supervision unquestionably alter the final prognosis.

2.8 Burden of Illness for Patient and Carer

For the individual, dementia presents a number of challenges that can undoubtedly lead to various negative emotions and which can impact on quality of life. The challenges are diverse and may alter throughout the course of the illness: frustration at memory failures, loss of self-esteem and confidence, mood disorder and agitated behaviours. Gauging the extent of these problems has traditionally relied on direct observation and carer proxy reports. Yet, the illness experience when persons with dementia are questioned directly may not reflect with the same severity the descriptions of suffering relayed by carers and assumptions made by society in general (de Boer et al. 2007; Steeman et al. 2007).

With the exception of the earliest stages of dementia, insight into the person's own predicament is generally poor. Defining outcomes such as health-related quality of life has only recently begun to be explored. This has led to the development of several dementia-specific quality of life instruments that are applicable in different stages of the disease (Ettema et al. 2005; Ettema et al. 2007). In the early and midstages, self-report instruments are recommended, while in later stages observation scales can be used (Schölzel-Dorenbos et al. 2007). How best to assess the subjective perceptions and experiences of the person with dementia in later stages of the disease in a reliable and convincing way remains as yet unclear.

It is accepted that those caring for persons with dementia are placed under significant strain. The level of burden is generally higher than other caregiver groups (González-Salvador et al. 1999). Caregiver burden is driven by several factors. The factors may be intrinsic to the carer, like carer age, gender, coping skills, or extrinsic factors that reflect the characteristics of the person with dementia. Higher caregiver burden is reported where the person with dementia is a spouse, older, or more functionally or behaviourally impaired. Another extrinsic example is the social milieu, with the burden related to the extent of external support and provision of respite opportunities.

2.9 Management of Dementia

It is important to address the everyday needs and wants of persons with dementia who for various reasons are disempowered but who may have reasonable concerns relating to safety, forgetfulness, communication or indeed everyday pursuits involving leisure activities that all warrant attention (Brodaty et al. 2003).

General care and psychosocial measures are the mainstay of care management. Education, psychological support, engagement with social services and charitable groups are all recommended but are necessarily problematic for those individuals living alone and without insight or an immediate advocate. The needs of the carer(s) become increasingly relevant as the disease progresses. In general therefore, combined support programmes, focused on the needs of both the person with dementia and the carer, are more effective than single support for patient or carer (Dröes et al. 2004). Issues related to driving, finance and placement create frequent challenges.

Specific pharmacological therapies are licensed for use in dementia (memantine) and more specifically AD (drugs known as "cholinesterase inhibitors"). Their effect is limited but may in some instances partly ameliorate the severity of cognitive symptoms and provide several months of clinical benefit. Secondary symptoms such as depression may require specific drug use. Pharmacotherapy should act in tandem with, and not replace, psychosocial interventions.

Tying together the various facets of multidisciplinary care and monitoring the process in the individual person and his carer are vital and often require the interest and commitment of a case manager. This could be a primary care physician, psychiatrist or elderly care specialist working in conjunction with specialist nursing and care management staff.

References

Alzheimer, A. (1907) Uber eine eigenartige Erkrankung der Hirnrinde. Allgemeine Zeitschrift für Psychiatrie und Psychisch-Gerichtliche Medizin, 64:146–148.

Berchtold, N.C., Cotman, C.W. (1998) Evolution in the conceptualization of dementia and Alzheimer's disease: Greco-Roman period to the 1960s. Neurobiology Aging, 19:173–189.

Brodaty, H., Green, A., Koschera, A. (2003) Meta-analysis of psychosocial interventions for caregivers of people with dementia. Journal of the American Geriatrics Society, 51: 657–664.

Craig, D., Mirakhur, A., Hart, D.J., McIlroy, S.P., Passmore, A.P. (2005) A cross-sectional study of neuropsychiatric symptoms in 435 patients with Alzheimer's disease. The American Journal of Geriatric Psychiatry, 13:460–468.

de Boer, M.E., Hertogh, C.M., Dröes, R.M., Riphagen, I.I., Jonker, C., Eefsting, J.A. (2007) Suffering from dementia – the patient's perspective: A review of the literature. International Psychogeriatrics, 19:1021–1039.

Dröes, R.M., Goffin, J.J.M., Breebaart, E., de Rooij, E., Vissers, H., Bleeker, J.A.C., van Tilburg, W. (2004) Support programmes for caregivers of people with dementia: A review of methods and effects. In: B. Miesen, G. Jones (eds.) Care-Giving in Dementia III. Routledge, UK, pp. 214–239.

Ettema, T.P., Dröes, R.M., de Lange, J., Mellenbergh, G.J., Ribbe, M.W. (2005) A review of quality of life instruments used in dementia. Quality of Life Research, 14:675–686.

Ettema, T.P., Dröes, R.M., de Lange, J., Mellenbergh, G.J., Ribbe, M.W. (2007) QUALIDEM: Development and evaluation of a dementia specific quality of life instrument-validation. International Journal of Geriatric Psychiatry, 22:424–430.

Fratiglioni, L., Launer, L.J., Andersen, K., Breteler, M.M., Copeland, J.R., Dartigues, J.F., Lobo, A., Martinez-Lage, J., Soininen, H., Hofman, A. (2000) Incidence of dementia and major subtypes in Europe: A collaborative study of population-based cohorts (Neurologic Diseases in the Elderly Research Group). Neurology, 54:S10–S15.

González-Salvador, M.T., Arango, C., Lyketsos, C.G., Barba, A.C. (1999) The stress and psychological morbidity of the Alzheimer patient caregiver. International Journal of Geriatric Psychiatry, 14:701–710.

Hofman, A., Rocca, W.A., Brayne, C., Breteler, M.M., Clarke, M., Cooper, B., Copeland, J.R., Dartigues, J.F., da Silva Droux, A., Hagnell, O. et al. (1991) The prevalence of dementia in Europe: A collaborative study of 1980–1990 findings. Eurodem Prevalence Research Group. International Journal of Epidemiology, 20:736–748.

Jameson, T. (1811) Essays on the Changes of the Human Body and Its Different Ages. J.G. Bernard, London.

Jönsson, L., Berr, C. (2005) Cost of dementia in Europe. European Journal of Neurology, 12: 50–53.

Lobo, A., Launer, L.J., Fratiglioni, L., Andersen, K., Di Carlo, A., Breteler, M.M., Copeland, J.R., Dartigues, J.F., Jagger, C., Martinez-Lage, J., Soininen, H., Hofman, A. (2000) Prevalence of dementia and major subtypes in Europe: A collaborative study of population-based cohorts (Neurologic Diseases in the Elderly Research Group). Neurology, 54:S4–S9.

Schölzel-Dorenbos, C.J., Ettema, T.P., Bos, J., Boelens-van der Knoop, E., Gerritsen, D.L., Hoogeveen, F., de Lange, J., Meihuizen, L., Dröes, R.M. (2007) Evaluating the outcome of interventions on quality of life in dementia: Selection of the appropriate scale. International Journal of Geriatric Psychiatry, 22:511–519.

Steeman, E., Godderis, J., Grypdonck, M., De Bal, N., Dierckx de Casterlé, B. (2007) Living with dementia from the perspective of older people: Is it a positive story? Aging and Mental Health, 11:119–130.

Werner, P., Korczyn, A.D. (2008) Mild cognitive impairment: Conceptual, assessment, ethical, and social issues. Clinical Interventions in Aging, 3:413–420.

Wimo, A., Winblad, B. (2008) Economical aspects of dementia. Handbook of Clinical Neurology, 89:137–146.

Chapter 3
State of the Art in Electronic Assistive Technologies for People with Dementia

Ricardo Castellot Lou, Angele Giuliano, and Maurice D. Mulvenna

Abstract It is estimated by 2050 that one-third of Europe's population will be over 60. Life expectancy has on average already risen by 2.5 years per decade and the number of old people aged 80+ is expected to grow by 180%. Nowadays, there are 5.5 million cases of Alzheimer-afflicted people in Europe and more new cases being added every year. In fact Alzheimer's disease has been called the "plague of the twenty-first century". There is currently no cure for this disease; however, prevention and early diagnosis may play a huge role in delaying the onset of the worst effects of this severe disease. Modern technologies could have an important role to satisfy main needs of people with dementia. Nonetheless, despite recent advancements in information and communication technologies and growing sales numbers, industry has been rather reluctant to standardise access technologies and to implement them in a "Design for All approach". Because of this, in last years, there have been launched in Europe a great number of initiatives, both public and private, which try to improve the situation of those persons who suffer this ailment and that will be detailed in this chapter.

Abbreviations

AAL	Ambient Assisting Living
EMA	Electronic Memory Aid
FP5	Fifth Framework Programme
GPRS	General Packet Radio Service
GPS	Global Positioning System
GSM	Global System for Mobile communications
ICT	Information and Communication Technology
IR	Infra Red
IST	Information Society Technology
PDA	Personal Digital Assistant

R.C. Lou (✉)
Telefonica I+D, Parque Tecnológico Walqa – Ed. 1, 22197, Cuarte (Huesca), Spain
e-mail: rcl@tid.es

M.D. Mulvenna, C.D. Nugent (eds.), *Supporting People with Dementia Using Pervasive Health Technologies*, Advanced Information and Knowledge Processing, DOI 10.1007/978-1-84882-551-2_3, © Springer-Verlag London Limited 2010

3.1 Introduction

There is a vast range of associations and companies along the EU (European Alzheimer's Associations 2009) that are offering some kind of support for persons with dementia and their carers. Most of them are informational websites that offer helpful information for carers, but seem less attuned to the persons with dementia and furthermore they do not offer personalised content. Information and Communication Technology (ICT) solutions, aimed at compensating for deficiencies such as memory problems and inconsistent daily activities, demonstrate that people with mild to moderate dementia are capable of handling simple electronic equipment and can benefit from it in terms of acquiring more confidence and feeling more positive (Reinersmann et al. 2007). Major ICT support for coping with behavioural and psychological changes in dementia is relatively disregarded as yet, while support for social contact can be effectively realised through the new technologies that are appearing on the market every day.

Some of the needs, that people with dementia and their informal carers currently perceive as insufficiently met by regular care and support services, can be alleviated, or even be met, using modern Information and Communication Technology.

However, most often, the design and the implementation of appliances, mobile phones and remote controls are driven by the ambition to satisfy users that are already engaged in modern technologies. Thus many people with disabilities, in particular persons with cognitive disabilities and older persons, are excluded from using modern technologies, at home and in the public. I2Home (2009) and MORE (2009), two projects involved in making life easier for persons with any disability, have considered these aspects and have focused their work in developing accessible and easy to use home appliances and devices for elderly and disabled people. Their main objective is that these persons are not severely impeded any longer in participating in our society, in living an independent life and in realising their full potential.

However, despite all these new initiatives, support for carers continues being urgently needed and governments have a key role to play in raising awareness and improving outcomes for sufferers of dementia and those around them. Significant resources will be required to address the clinical and social aspects of Alzheimer's disease as well as new models of care that span across health and social services are needed (Fig. 3.1).

Based on those unmet needs that were most frequently mentioned by a group of people with dementia and their carers that participated in a field research (Reinersmann et al. 2007), we can pick out four main strands: the need for support with regard to symptoms of dementia (the most frequent one being the loss of memory), the need for social contact and company, the need of supporting daily life activities and the need for health monitoring and perceived safety.

The need for general and personalised information mentioned by persons with dementia refers to information on the diagnosis, condition, available support services and care (including information on support for memory problems). Informal carers want information on diagnosis, prognosis, treatment, care structures, day care

Fig. 3.1 Person with
dementia and her carer

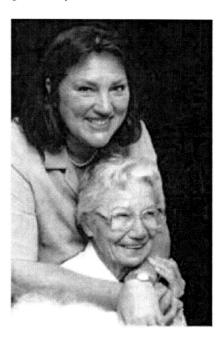

facilities and other services including legal and financial issues. The mentioned need for support with regard to symptoms of dementia refers to all types of instrumental support in a person's daily life activities, including support to enhance participation and supervision/guidance.

The need for social contact and company refers specifically to ways of staying connected with family, friends and the social environment and also to feeling useful. Reported needs for health monitoring and perceived safety refer to the wish to be cared for and to feel safe when the disease progresses and disabilities increase.

3.2 Support for Memory

To help Persons with dementia undertake specific types of time-linked tasks (e.g. taking medication, keeping appointments or following a daily schedule) various possibilities of automatic reminders via Electronic Memory Aids (EMAs) are explored, such as NeuroPage (2009) and MemoJog (2009) solutions. The first one is the most common and simple since it only uses an ordinary pager and that can be an advantage because of its easy use. The second one makes use of the new generation of mobile phones and palmtop computing technologies to provide memory jogging messages to the user about upcoming activities for the day. In this respect, COGKNOW (2009) also offers several memory services that not only help Alzheimer's patients in their daily life activities but also provides them enjoyment and comfort as well as ways to support their independence and communication with other people (Fig. 3.2).

Fig. 3.2 Electronic memory aid

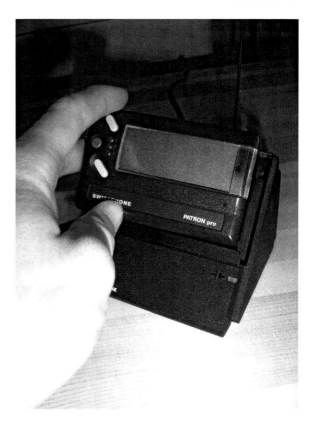

Most researchers recognise the importance of involving informal carers in the implementation of EMAs, since carers motivate the person with dementia to use the EMA but also benefit themselves, as use of an EMA by a person with dementia reduces feelings of worry in the informal carer. An EMA informing the person verbally, using vocal recordings, of specific appointments or tasks, also has positive effects on Alzheimer patients.

Besides training the dementia patients' brain and stimulating their memory with solutions as Smartbrain (2009) system, which not only stimulates but also develops the main cognitive capacities of adult people by training their memory, language, calculation and orientation, several services present in the market also consider relaxation and enjoyment as other important activities in the daily life of Alzheimer-afflicted people. COGKNOW has taken these aspects into account and not only centres on memory assistance or help for daily activities such as eating, but has implemented functions that focus on enriching the life of persons with dementia. One of these implemented functions is a music library that can be played by patients whenever they want to. This service stimulates them and improves their feelings of comfort and happiness since in many studies researches suggest that music can have a strong effect on mental stability of people with dementia (Yasuda et al. 2006).

3.3 Support for Daily Life Activities

Most of the people with dementia live in the community and are supported by both family and friends and professional carers and services. A minority lives in institutions such as homes for the elderly, sheltered housing projects and nursing homes. Caring for a relative with Alzheimer's disease has been described as "life changing, exhausting and stressful". To help people in this matter, several initiatives, such as Proyecto Alzheimer (2009) or Enabling Smart Houses (2009), have been carried out in the EU. The first one consists of a social and healthy approach that tries to face the consequences that Alzheimer's disease provokes in both sufferers and relatives. The project focuses on a residence for Alzheimer's sufferers coupled with an investigation and provision of training about the disease making this centre stand out among the several other centres that have been built.

Designing and developing smart home technologies that could assist dementia sufferers within their own living environment is another important aspect that both patients and carers point out as essential to carry a normal life. Enabling Smart Houses has considered this and the house itself monitors the occupant's behaviour and, through automatic equipment and verbal prompts and reminders, also reacts to any issues that arise. Other projects and initiatives available on the market, such as Easy Line Plus (2009), not only consider these aspects in making easier and more comfortable the normal life of Alzheimer patients, but also take into account the need for compatibility and development of devices close to market. Good ICT design is highly important and can add value to the offered product/s (Fig. 3.3).

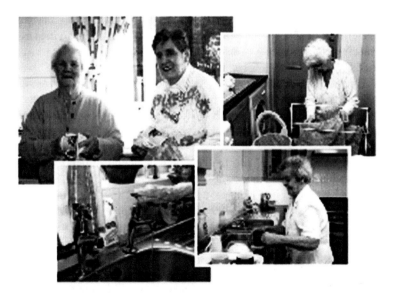

Fig. 3.3 Persons with dementia daily life activities

People are more and more concerned about losing their independence at some point in their lives, be it through growing older, becoming ill or disabled. Organisations that support people living at home need to provide a safe environment and be certain that the right services are provided at the right time. Fortunately, nowadays there are many different technologies and appliances specially designed and adapted to those needs. Patients can also buy many of these devices independently. Companies such as Tunstall (2009) or Alares (2009) have on offer different services or products especially developed to enhance a person's independence, health and feeling of well-being. People who need some kind of support can buy devices that will help them avoid emergency situations inside and outside home, but before doing so, they should contact their local social services authority or similar support departments.

Unfortunately, specialised support is not growing at the same high rate as the elder population numbers and this makes necessary the development of technological systems, such as COGKNOW, to give sufficient assistance. This highlights the situation that there are not enough products and services oriented to healthcare and life improvement of patients who suffer from Alzheimer. Nonetheless, although not specifically designed for dementia patients, there are European projects and systems developed to improve the life of persons with disabilities. In this way we find projects such as ALADIN (2009), INHOME (2009), MonAMI (2009), OLDES (2009) or SHARE-it (2009) which correspond to the European Information Society Technology (IST) Thematic Priority in the framework of Ambient Assisting Living (AAL) for the Ageing Society. They mainly focus on elderly people and the improvement of their quality of life. Intelligent home environments, assistive systems and the development of generic technologies for managing the domestic environment are some of the facilities that projects mentioned above offer to elderly. These could be also used by Alzheimer's sufferers since some of their needs are similar to the elderly people's ones: support for memory, daily life activities assistance and enhancing feelings of safety inside and outside home.

ENABLE (2009), "Enabling technologies for persons with dementia", was one of the first European longitudinal studies inside the Fifth Framework Programme for Research and Innovation (FP5) which investigated whether it is possible to facilitate independent living and promote well-being of persons with dementia living in their own home through access to products which allow them to carry out their daily life activities. Spanning across five countries, (Norway, Finland, Ireland, the UK and Lithuania), a total of 140 families with dementia sufferers were recruited to the study, which involved the testing out of assistive technologies in their homes. The products introduced into people's homes included an automatic night-and-day calendar, a gas cooker monitor, an automatic night lamp, a picture button telephone and an item locator. From all of these products, only two (the night-and-day calendar and the picture telephone) are now available commercially and are supplied by providers in Sweden and Norway.

COGKNOW also considers all these services and helps Alzheimer's patients in their daily life activities providing them contentment and comfort, ways to support their memory and to enhance communication with other people. However, although

COGKNOW does not consider all services in the same way like ENABLE the final result is similar – providing the same utilities and help services. Likewise, another system called PEAT (2009) provides queuing and scheduling assistance for individuals with memory, attention and cognitive disorders. With this system, persons suffering from this impairment can feel safe and calm, an important aspect that a lot of experts highlight as essential, since it also provides a virtual caregiver presence 24 h a day via cellular phones.

3.4 Support for Social Contacts

Continuing in the same vein and as we have already mentioned, people with dementia have many needs during the progression of their disease, varying from memory support in mild dementia, to support in almost all aspects of daily functioning in severe dementia. Family carers, neighbours and friends meet some of these needs, while professional carers meet others. However, despite the efforts of these informal and formal carers, not all the needs of people with dementia can be met. The reasons for this include the limited time that both informal and formal carers can give to the person with dementia, and the lack of, or limited availability of, professional services attuned specifically to the concrete needs of individual people with dementia.

With respect to support for social contacts, some authors (White and Dorman 2000) analysed the contents of messages posted on an Alzheimer mailing group and concluded that the opportunity to share, unburden or vent, is perceived as empowering and helpful to carers. Almost every Alzheimer association offers a website where people with dementia and their carers can join forums, post messages or chat with fellow sufferers. Many Alzheimer associations also have a 24-h telephone support service for emotional support and information on regional support services like Alzheimer café's and meeting centres.

In 2003, another study suggested that with the use of multimedia as a source of reminiscence, patients could exhibit more control of the direction of the conversation. A touch-screen display was developed to convey photographs, video or music, and it was also compared to traditional reminiscence methods. As a result of this study, the patients using the multimedia system showed stronger and more prolonged engagement during the conversations (Fig. 3.4).

Through several other studies, such as "Televisits", contact between elderly people living in a nursing home and their family via videophone was demonstrated to promote social contact. In a similar study, Sävenstedt and others (2003) showed that a videophone as a means of communication between patient and family reduced feelings of guilt in family members, allowed more frequent visits than was possible with face-to-face visits and let family members see the physical and emotional state of the patient on a daily basis. In some cases the conversations were more focused and of better quality than during face-to-face visits. In most cases, however, more emphasis was placed on the family member to direct and lead the conversations which was seen by many as demanding. The relationship between staff and family

Fig. 3.4 People with
dementia can feel better if
they can maintain social
contact

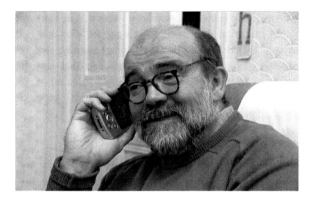

members improved as a side effect of staff helping the patient use the videophone.
These are some of the results that ACTION (2009), a videophone service for frail
older persons who prefer to stay and live in their own homes but who are in need
of support from nurses and relatives, has extracted after performing tests. Family
carers feel safer and more competent in their role of caring and the older people and
their relatives develop informal support networks with other families more readily
and with greater ease.

Internet-based applications designed to provide carers with clinical, decision-
making and emotional support were evaluated in field trials and the preliminary
results showed the system to be beneficial both to carers and people with dementia. As a consequence of that, several European projects (SOPRANO (SOPRANO
2009), TeleCARE (TeleCARE 2009)) and other private systems (doc@home
(doc@home 2009), SafetyNet (SafetyNet 2009)) have been designed in order to
provide a systematic approach to the management of the care of patients with long-
term conditions or chronic diseases in their own homes and other locations remote
from the clinicians' office. Besides this, these solutions also enable the provision
of flexible individualised and supportive services and healthcare in order to promote independent living and integration of people with functional impairments into
social life.

3.5 Enhancing Feeling of Safety

However, enhancing Alzheimer patients' feelings of safety might be the main essential area most frequently mentioned as unmet by both sufferers and their carers
since they can live in a normal way, maintaining their contacts and doing their
daily activities more easily and calmly if they feel safe. With regard to this matter,
beneficial effects of computer systems have been observed on orientation, feelings of anxiety and independency in patients suffering from Alzheimer's disease.
Besides this, implementing monitoring technologies and detection devices or alarm
systems inside and outside the home of elderly persons is potentially useful to

enhance (perceived) safety and security of the person suffering from dementia as well as carers. Over the last few decades, detections devices and alarm systems have been developed for different Alzheimer's associations. Investigation and diagnostic groups have been focusing on protecting patients from dangers such as fires, gas leaks and floods with such devices. COGKNOW shares this principle in making use of several sensors and alarms that notify to the tenant if something goes wrong in the house. As a consequence of this and since COGKNOW is specifically designed to solve and help mild dementia patients, these people could find in this project an appropriate and satisfactory service.

Nowadays scientists and researchers are becoming more aware about the problems suffered by people with dementia. For that reason, several systems were and are already being developed as well with the purpose of helping these persons in emergency situations using ambient and unobtrusive devices. This is the case of EMERGE (2009) and SAFE21 (2009); two projects financed by the European Commission, which aim to develop a solution that provides early assistance to the patient, and build on existing social alarms that provide an emergency response to a call initiated by a user, respectively.

The non-interference with the daily life activities of the dementia sufferer is, as we mentioned before, a very important aspect which should be taken into account in the development of new help systems. In that way, a straying prevention system that can counteract Alzheimer's sufferers wandering was developed in 2006 (Lin et al. 2006). The system consists of indoor residence monitoring, outdoor activity monitoring, emergency rescue service and remote monitoring that can be accessed via a number of mobile devices such as a mobile phone, PDA, notebook or computer. The indoor monitor detects movement between certain areas within the home. Outdoor activities, accompanied or unaccompanied, are monitored in a pre-set activity area, which is activated by pressing a button on the location tracking device. Message or alarms, respectively, are generated and forwarded via Global System for Mobile communications (GSM) if the patient leaves the home environment or the activity area. In case of an emergency, the person with dementia can activate an emergency button which sends a message to the call centre where the situation, location and geographical information and location coordinates are analysed and relayed to care providers, search teams and family members. Conversely, through the secure remote monitoring facility included in the system, family members or care providers can also access patient's location information at any time by logging onto the system. In this way both relatives and carers will be able to be calmer and Alzheimer sufferers more independent and free (Fig. 3.5).

As was illustrated previously, current new technologies have also a remarkable role in being assistive carers. An example of that is found in a fully automatic multisensor system, composed of Infra Red (IR) sensors connected to a personal computer installed in a patient's room, which was evaluated by some authors (Chan et al. 2002). This smart tool system proved valid in assessing and recording data on activities such as getting out of bed, mobility and travel patterns of a psychotic patient with moderate cognitive decline and behavioural disorders.

Fig. 3.5 COGKNOW
personal digital assistant

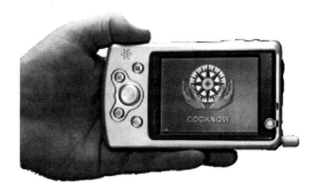

Besides all of this, in 2005, applying a user-driven design approach, a smart home environment consisting of different services and devices that aimed to assist people with dementia in various areas was developed and evaluated (Orpwood et al. 2005). During the night, for example, a lighting system was activated if a patient had left the bed. On returning to bed the lights would fade off after a few minutes. However, failure to return to bed after a pre-defined period of time would result in the communication system telling the patient that it is night time and they should not go to the exit during the night and verbally remind them to return to bed. In addition to the night monitoring, the system incorporated a cooking monitor service, which detected problems and potential dangers during the cooking process. Although the cooker monitor was a very useful tool and during evaluations this device worked well, it caused some irritation to users when the cooker was turned off under false positive situations. This situation disclosed that every system developed to help Alzheimer's sufferers had to take into account not only their possible oversights but also their feeling of independence and control of the situation.

Alzheimer disease mainly affects memory and mental functioning (e.g. thinking and speaking), but it can also lead to other problems such as confusion, changes of mood and disorientation in time and space. According to this last matter, in a study comparing four biomechanical activity devices to index wandering, Algase and others (2003) found the Step Watch particularly able to assess the amount and daily course of wandering behaviour in people with dementia. In this context, boundary alarms (activated by a wristband) or electronic tagging with bracelets and monitoring stations were found to be effective, reliable and successful in detecting wandering as well as reducing patient and carer stress. This is the intention of some products such as SIMAP (2009), GPS Columba (2009) or Keruve (2009), which make use of small, portable and discreet devices implementing new GPS technology in order to locate the person anywhere and all the time. A bedside monitoring system was also tested in a hospital setting with three floor lighting about wandering detection. It relays an alarm to a personal handheld device alerting the carer so that the necessary intervention can be performed (Figs. 3.6 and 3.7).

Fig. 3.6 Columba GPS
bracelet

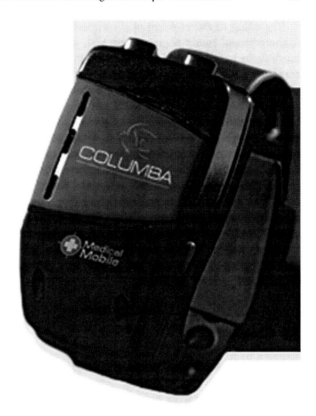

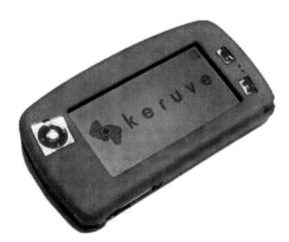

Fig. 3.7 Keruve locator for
Alzheimer disease persons

Regarding to the problem of disorientation, there are more help systems such as the personal handy phone system that, worn by the patient as a pendant, could transmit the patient's position with an accuracy of 60 m to a personal computer. The computer generates a map of the area, and then automatically sends this map via e-mail to the carer who can view it on a mobile phone.

On the other hand, COGKNOW not only considers all these aspects, but also takes into account the possibility of showing the way back home to the wandered person. Carrying a Personal Digital Assistant (PDA), Alzheimer's patients could be located everywhere at any time as long as, besides Global Positioning System (GPS) that indicates the position on the PDA, information can be sent to a server using any kind of data communication such as General Packet Radio Service (GPRS). Patients could also use the GPS to go to the place they want or even be helped by making a call to the emergency contact since the PDA has implemented GSM technology as well. Besides all of these technologies currently available, COGKNOW looks at the future making its PDA a multipurpose device, which will be able to implement new technologies in an easy and simple way, allowing giving better attention to Alzheimer's patients' problems.

3.6 Conclusion

To conclude with this chapter and, after revising the principal technologies and ways for helping people who suffer mild dementia, we can say that there are many products, devices and services available in the market which can make the life of those persons easier as well as help carers and family members to take care of them. However, and despite all big efforts for covering most of Alzheimer's sufferers needs, these people cannot find a service capable of helping them with their daily activities at the same time that it reinforces their memory, enhances their feeling of safety and maintains their social contacts. That is the objective of COGKNOW system. All the devices integrated in its architecture cover and settle the needs shown in many studies of Alzheimer's patients. Moreover, COGKNOW also uses all the current industry standards and available technologies, which turn it into a solution of great potential value and help for people who suffer this ailment.

References

ACTION. (2009) http://www.actionservice.se/EngDefault.htm . Accessed 14 January 2009.
ALADIN. (2009) http://www.ambient-lighting.eu /. Accessed 14 January 2009.
Alares. (2009), http://www.alares.es . Accessed 14 January 2009.
Algase, D.L., Beattie, E.R.A., Leitsch, S.A., Beel-Bates, C.A. (2003) Biomechanical activity devices to index wandering behaviour in dementia. American Journal of Alzheimer's Disease and Other Dementias, 18(2):85–92. doi: 10.1177/153331750301800202.
Chan, M., Campo, E., Laval, E., Estève, D. (2002) Validation of a remote monitoring system for the elderly: Application to mobility measurements. Technology and Health Care, 10(5): 391–399.

COGKNOW. (2009) http://www.cogknow.eu /. Accessed 14 January 2009.
doc@home.   (2009)   http://www.docobo.co.uk/ArticlePage.aspx?articleId=6&topParentId=7.
    Accessed 14 January 2009.
Easy Line Plus. (2009) http://www.arenque-ks.com/easynet/potencialimpact.html. Accessed 14
    January 2009.
EMERGE. (2009) http://www.emerge-project.eu/. Accessed 14 January 2009.
ENABLE. (2009) http://www.enable-project.eu/. Accessed 14 January 2009.
Enabling Smart Houses. (2009) http://www.bath.ac.uk/bime/projects/dc_projects.htm. Accessed
    14 January 2009.
European   Alzheimer's   Associations.   (2009)   http://www.alzheimer-europe.org/?content=
    findmorehelp&engine=assoc. Accessed 14 January 2009.
GPS Columba. (2009) http://en.eu.medicalmobile.com/iiix/home/. Accessed 14 January 2009.
I2Home. (2009) http://www.i2home.org/. Accessed 14 January 2009.
INHOME. (2009) http://www.ist-inhome.eu/. Accessed 14 January 2009.
Keruve. (2009). http://www.keruve.com/. Accessed 14 January 2009.
Lin, C.C., Chiu, M.J., Hsiao, C.C., Lee, R.G., Tsai, Y.S. (2006) Wireless health care service sys-
    tem for elderly with dementia. IEEE Transactions on Information Technology in Biomedicine,
    10(4):696–704. doi: 10.1109/TITB.2006.874196.
MemoJog. (2009) http://www.computing.dundee.ac.uk/projects/memojog/. Accessed 14 January
    2009.
MonAMI. (2009) http://www.monami.info/. Accessed 14 January 2009.
MORE. (2009) http://www.is.tuwien.ac.at/fortec/reha.e/projects/more/more.html. Accessed 14
    January 2009.
NeuroPage. (2009). http://www.neuropage.nhs.uk/. Accessed 14 January 2009.
OLDES. (2009). http://www.oldes.eu/. Accessed 14 January 2009.
Orpwood, R., Gibbs, C., Adlam, T., Faulkner, R., Meegahawatte, D. (2005) The design of smart
    homes for people with dementia – user interface aspects. Universal Access in the Information
    Society, 4(2):156–164. doi: 10.1007/s10209-005-0120-7.
PEAT. (2009) http://www.brainaid.com/. Accessed 14 January 2009.
Proyecto Alzheimer. (2009) http://www.fundacionreinasofia.es/proyectoalzheimer/visita-nueva/
    proyecto-ides-idweb.html. Accessed 14 January 2009.
Reinersmann, A., Lauriks, S., van der Roest, H.G., Meiland, F.J.M., Davies, R.J., Moelaert,
    F., Mulvenna, M.D., Nugent, C.D., Dröes, R.M. (2007) Review of ICT-based services for
    identified unmet needs in people with dementia. Ageing Research Reviews, 6(3): 223–246.
SAFE21. (2009) http://www.pricepartnership.com/safe21/home.htm. Accessed 14 January 2009.
SafetyNet. (2009) http://www.createabilityinc.com/safetynet_info.html. Accessed 14 January
    2009.
Sävenstedt, S., Brulin, C., Sandman, P.O. (2003) Family members' narrated experiences of com-
    municating via video-phone with patients with dementia staying at a nursing home. Journal of
    Telemedicine and Telecare, 9(4):216–220. doi: 10.1258/135763303322225544.
SHARE-it. (2009) http://www.ist-shareit.eu/shareit/welcome-to-share-it. Accessed 14 January
    2009.
SIMAP. (2009) http://www.simapglobal.com/. Accessed 14 January 2009.
Smartbrain. (2009) http://www.smartbrain.net. Accessed 14 January 2009.
SOPRANO. (2009) http://www.soprano-ip.org/. Accessed 14 January 2009.
TeleCARE. (2009) http://www.uninova.pt/~telecare/. Accessed 14 January 2009.
Tunstall. (2009) http://www.tunstall.co.uk/. Accessed 14 January 2009.
White, M.H., Dorman, S.M. (2000) Online support for caregivers: Analysis of an internet
    Alzheimer mail-group. Computers in Nursing, 18(4):168–176.
Yasuda, K., Beckman, B., Yoneda, M., Yoneda, H., Iwamoto, A., Nakamura, T. (2006) Successful
    guidance by automatic output of music and verbal messages for daily behavioural distur-
    bances of three individuals with dementia. Neuropsychological Rehabilitation, 16(1):66–82.
    doi: 10.1080/09602010443000191.

Chapter 4
Review of ICT-Based Services for Identified Unmet Needs in People with Dementia

Steve Lauriks, Annika Reinersmann, Henriëtte Geralde van der Roest,
Franka Meiland, Richard Davies, Ferial Moelaert, Maurice D. Mulvenna,
Chris D. Nugent, and Rose-Marie Dröes

Abstract Some of the needs that people with dementia and their informal carers currently perceive as insufficiently met by regular care and support services might be alleviated, or even be met, using modern Information and Communication Technology (ICT). The study described in this chapter was designed to provide an insight into the state of the art in ICT solutions that could contribute to meet the most frequently mentioned unmet needs by people with dementia and their informal carers. These needs can be summarized as (1) the need for general and personalized information; (2) the need for support with regard to symptoms of dementia; (3) the need for social contact and company; and (4) the need for health monitoring and perceived safety. Databases that were searched include PubMed, Cinahl, Psychinfo, Google (Scholar), INSPEC and IEEE. In total 22 websites and 46 publications were included that satisfied the following criteria: the article reports on people with dementia and/or their informal carers and discusses an ICT device that has been tested within the target group and has proven to be helpful. Within the first need area 18 relevant websites and three studies were included; within the second need area 4 websites and 20 publications were included. Within the third and fourth need area 11 and 12 publications were included, respectively. Most articles reported on uncontrolled studies. It is concluded that the informational websites offer helpful information for carers but seem less attuned to the person with dementia and do not offer personalized information. ICT solutions aimed at compensating for disabilities, such as memory problems and daily activities, demonstrate that people with mild to moderate dementia are capable of handling simple electronic equipment and can benefit from it in terms of more confidence and enhanced positive affect. Instrumental ICT support for coping with behavioural

S. Lauriks (✉)
Academic Department of Psychiatry, Regional Institute for Mental Health Services GGZ-Buitenamstel Geestgronden/EMGO-Institute, VU University Medical Center, Amsterdam, The Netherlands
e-mail: s.lauriks@gmail.com

This chapter is an abridged version of Lauriks et al. (2007).

M.D. Mulvenna, C.D. Nugent (eds.), *Supporting People with Dementia Using Pervasive Health Technologies*, Advanced Information and Knowledge Processing, DOI 10.1007/978-1-84882-551-2_4, © Springer-Verlag London Limited 2010

and psychological changes in dementia is relatively disregarded as yet, while support for social contact can be effectively realized through, for example, simplified
(mobile) phones or videophones or (entertainment) robots. GPS technology and
monitoring systems are proven to result in enhanced feelings of safety and less
fear and anxiety. Though these results are promising, more controlled studies in
which the developed ICT solutions are tested in real-life situations are needed
before implementing them in the care for people with dementia. It is recommended
that future studies also focus on the integration of the current techniques and
solutions.

4.1 Introduction

As the population in our society is ageing, the number of people with chronic diseases is growing. To serve this growing group in an effective and efficient way,
more specific knowledge of the needs of people with chronic diseases, as well as
of individual variations in needs within different groups of people with chronic disease, is required. One of these groups is people with dementia, whose numbers are
expected to double over the next two decades (Ferri et al. 2005). Most of the people
with dementia live in the community and are supported by family and friends and
professional carers and services. A minority live in institutions such as homes for
the elderly, sheltered housing projects and nursing homes (Health Council of the
Netherlands 2002; Ferri et al. 2005).

People with dementia have many needs during the progression of their disease,
varying from memory support in mild dementia to support in almost all aspects of
daily functioning in severe dementia. Family carers, neighbours and friends meet
some of these needs, while professional carers meet others. However, despite the
efforts of these informal and formal carers, not all the needs of people with dementia can be met. The reasons for this include the limited time that both informal
and formal carers have available, and the lack of, or limited availability of, professional services attuned specifically to the concrete needs of individual people with
dementia.

A recent gap analysis in two regions of The Netherlands (Amsterdam and
Nijmegen) showed that various types of services are available for all of the most frequently mentioned unmet needs (Dröes et al. 2005b). Several possible reasons were
mentioned to explain the fact that these needs are still perceived as unmet by people
with dementia and their carers. For example, patient and carer (or even professional
referrers) are not aware of the service offering that is available; they experience a
threshold for using professional services; there are mismatches between the way in
which services are offered and the individual needs of patients and/or carers. These
reasons are confirmed in the literature, where Coe and Neufeld (1999) conclude

that most people do not know where to go for help and that they have to take the initiative to find it. As one carer expresses "There is help if you just go after it. The help doesn't find you. You have to go after the help." (p. 575). Cox (1997) and Brodaty et al. (2005) reported that carers who did not use respite services felt they did not really need them, while Koffmann and Taylor (1997) observed that carers experienced guilt when letting their loved ones go into respite care. Also, Winslow (2003) describes barriers to service use, such as care receiver resistance, reluctance of the carer, hassles for the carer, concerns over quality and concerns over finances. Finally, the way in which the professional support is offered (intensity, frequency, flexibility, timing and location) does not always match the different individual needs (Koffmann and Taylor 1997; Gwyther 1998; Coe and Neufeld 1999; Perry and Bontinen 2001; Clare 2002). This often applies for standardized, and therefore non-flexible and non-personalized, care activities and programs. Biegel et al. (1993) found that people with dementia who do not use services or only in-home services were more functionally impaired and had inadequate informal support and more emotionally strained carers compared with users of out-of-home or both in- and out-of-home services. Coe and Neufeld (1999) describe the obstacles carers encounter when they have finally found the help they needed, "(...) for example, there was a delay in obtaining formal help, policies restricted the assistance that could be provided, and the application process was long and complex." (p. 575).

The need for more flexible, personalized care and support is fully in line with the emphasis in the literature for many years that individual needs of patients and carers can considerably differ because of a number of personal and contextual factors, such as the symptoms of the person with dementia, carer characteristics and utilized coping strategies, the relationship between the carer and the person with dementia, the support systems available to the carer and the perception of the quality of the relief that is offered (Duijnstee 1992; Dröes et al. 1996; Dunkin and Anderson-Hanley 1998; Burns 2000; Proctor and Testad 2005; Clare 2002).

Some of the needs that people with dementia and their informal carers currently perceive as insufficiently met by regular care and support services might be alleviated, or even be met, using modern Information and Communication Technology (ICT). In this chapter, we report on a review study that was aimed at getting insight into the state of the art of ICT solutions (in practice and research) that could contribute to meet these unmet needs of people with dementia and their informal carers. Based on the most frequently mentioned unmet needs by people with dementia and by their informal carers that were inventoried in field research among the target group (Dröes et al. 2006; Hancock et al. 2006; van der Roest et al. (2009), we focused our review study at the following need areas: (1) need for general and personalized information; (2) need for support with regard to symptoms of dementia; (3) need for social contact and company; and (4) need for health monitoring and perceived safety.

4.2 Method

4.2.1 Selection Criteria

Within the four selected areas of needs a further subdivision into more specific themes was made (see Table 4.1) based on concrete needs mentioned by people with dementia in these areas, as described in the literature (van der Roest et al. 2007) and in three recent field studies that identified both met and unmet needs in people with dementia and their informal and formal carers. Dröes et al. (2006) inventoried general needs with respect to quality of life among people with dementia who attend meeting centres and regular day care centres ($n = 106$) or who live in nursing homes ($n = 37$). Hancock et al. (2006) researched unmet needs of people with dementia ($n = 238$) in residential care using the Camberwell Assessment of Needs for the Elderly (CANE; Cummings et al. 1994). van der Roest et al. (2009)

Table 4.1 Studied need areas and themes

Needs areas	Specific themes
1. Need for general and personalized information	A. Information on dementia B. Information on service offerings C. Information on legal and financial issues and on care and support services D. Information on personal condition, care appointments and care planning
2. Need for support with regard to symptoms of dementia	A. ICT compensation for disabilities such as memory problems in daily life activities B. ICT supporting the carer, flexibly and personalized, in providing instrumental care to the person with dementia C. ICT support for people with dementia and carers regarding behavioural and psychological changes and how to cope with them D. Emotional support for patients and carers
3. The need for social contact and company for the person with dementia	Ways to stay connected with family, friends and the social environment and to be useful
4. The need for health monitoring and perceived safety for the person with dementia	The need to be cared for and to be safe when the disease progresses

conducted a large field study among 236 people with dementia living in the community and 322 carers using the Dutch version of the CANE (Dröes et al. 2004) and in-depth interviews.

From these studies it is clear that the need for general and personalized information mentioned by people with dementia refers to information on the diagnosis, condition, available support services (including information on support, for example, memory problems) and care appointments. Informal carers want information on diagnosis, prognosis, treatment, care structures, day care facilities and other services including legal and financial issues. The mentioned need for support with regard to symptoms of dementia refers to all types of instrumental support in daily life activities, including support to participate in activities and supervision/guidance.

The need for social contact and company refers specifically to ways of staying connected with family, friends and the social environment and to feel useful. Reported needs for health monitoring and perceived safety refer to the wish to be cared for and to feel secure when the disease progresses and disabilities increase.

For this review we focused on articles that were published before 15 November 2006 and met the following inclusion criteria:

- the article reports on people with cognitive disabilities related to dementia and/or their informal carers
- the article discusses an ICT device or application that has been tested within the target group
- the ICT device reported on in the article has proven to be helpful for the person with cognitive disabilities related to dementia and/or the informal carer on one of the selected needs areas of this review (see Table 4.1).

4.2.2 Search Procedure

We searched the following databases: PubMed, PsychInfo, Cinahl, INSPEC and IEEE. Besides that we searched on the Internet using Google Scholar. Within these searches we used a list of key words for each needs area (see Lauriks et al. 2007). The snowball effect furthermore enabled us to retrieve other publications based on the references in the publications found initially. The search procedure did not reveal information derived from unpublished studies.

4.2.3 Analysis

The searches within the mentioned databases initially resulted in 165 publications and websites. The analysis was performed by two groups of researchers: the first group consisted of three people with expertize in the clinical domain (AR, SL, RMD); the second group consisted of two people with expertize in information and communication technology (RJD, MDM). All articles were independently assessed with regard to the inclusion criteria by two researchers and compared afterwards.

In case of discrepancies the articles were considered again until consensus was reached. This resulted in 22 (examples of) relevant websites and 46 articles that satisfied the inclusion criteria for this review. The selected articles were analysed with regard to needs area, research sample and research design, functionality of the ICT solution/device and outcome or results for the target group (for detailed descriptions of the results of these analyses see Lauriks et al. 2007). The content of the selected ICT solutions and devices is described briefly in Section 4.3.

4.3 Results

4.3.1 Need for General and Personalized Information

In this needs area 18 relevant websites and three publications were found that satisfied the inclusion criteria.

4.3.1.1 Information on Dementia

Larner (2003) demonstrated that the use of the Internet by people with cognitive disorders and their carers is common and may increase involvement of patients in supervising and documenting their own health care.

The websites of Alzheimer associations provide digital information on dementia (e.g. www.alzheimer-europe.org or www.alz.org). Apart from prevalence figures, research information and advice on the practical, social and emotional consequences of the disease, some of these sites offer the opportunity to chat with fellow patients and carers (e.g. www.alzheimer-nederland.nl). A few sites include an informative section for people with dementia themselves (e.g. www.alz.co.uk).

As part of the UK's Alzheimer's Society project "Learning to Live with Dementia", Freeman et al. (2005) set up guidelines for accessible writing and web design for people with mild to moderate dementia. In order to attune (online) text to the needs of people with dementia they designed and evaluated a website in close collaboration with the target users, which improved the accessibility of the website.

The University of Florida provides a specialized website (www.alzonline.net) where carers are offered information on dementia as well as Internet- and telephone-based support and education. The Alzheimer Research Forum (www.alzforum.org) includes detailed information on clinical guidelines, the medical workup, drugs and non-pharmacological therapies for health care professionals, researchers and lay people.

4.3.1.2 Information on Service Offerings

Besides printed guides containing an overview of health care and welfare services, recently online "social charts" have become available in several European countries. They provide detailed information on national or regional services for professionals and/or specific patient groups. Social charts are offered by different organizations and therefore vary with regard to target users, ease-of-use and completeness. Some popular Dutch social charts are provided by the National Institute for Public Health and Environment (RIVM: www.kiesbeter.nl), the Trade organization of regional consumer- and patient-interest organizations (www.zorgbelang-nederland.nl) and the National society of informal and voluntary carers (MEZZO; www.mantelzorg.nl). The site www.hulpgids.nl focuses on mental health care and contains a database of over 1,200 clinicians, therapists and psychiatrists. More general sites (e.g. www.vraagwijzer.nl and www.2zw-adreswijzer.nl) offer information on health care, welfare, housing, social security, income, education and policy to a broad audience.

Social charts in other countries, such as www.desocialekaart.be in Belgium, www.alzonline.net in the state of Florida and www.aahsa.org in the USA, are in essence not very different, though some, like www.healthfinder.gov, also provide visitors with comprehensive information on the quality of care.

The social charts discussed above are typically quite static, generic (not specifically intended for people with dementia or their carers) and mainly provide a, often incomplete, list of addresses for services in the region. Personalized, context-sensitive and demand-orientated sites which exist for other diagnostics groups (e.g. www.voorlichtingopmaat.nl for rheumatism patients or www.stoppain.org for pain patients) are lacking for people with dementia and their informal carers.

4.3.1.3 Information on Legal and Financial Issues and on Care and Support Services

The websites of ministries responsible for public health, like the Dutch Ministry of Public Health, Welfare and Sports (VWS), offer information on financial issues, legislation, health insurance and other subjects related to financial and legal developments in care and support services (www.denieuwezorgverzekering.nl or www.minvws.nl). With the website www.zorgvoorbeter.nl, which is part of a national action program, the Dutch Ministry of VWS aims to improve quality of care in home care and institutional care for the elderly and disabled by providing transparency, quality indicators and stimulating improvement trajectories in health care organizations. The site also offers descriptions and examples of high-quality care for people with dementia. A telephone service (the "Mantelzorglijn") offers support to informal carers and can also be contacted for legal and financial advice with regard to care and support services.

4.3.1.4 Information on Personal Condition, Care Appointments and Care Planning

In the USA, the Geisinger Health System with its "MyChart" application allows patients to communicate electronically with their medical care providers and view selected portions of their Electronic Health Record (EHR) (Hassol et al. 2004). Likewise, the Henry Ford Hospital in Detroit, Michigan has over 50,000 patients using an application called "MyHealth" to view customized health information, obtain lab test results and renew prescriptions online (www.henryford.com).

Recently, a new system called the Patient Access Electronic Record System (PAERS) was trailed in the UK, which allows patients visiting their General Practitioner (GP) to look up their health records and book in for their appointments (Honeyman et al. 2005). It is not reported whether people with dementia or their informal carers use this system.

Although EHRs are applied on a small scale in hospitals, home care organizations and GP networks in many European countries, patients and informal carers have no access to these records yet. As an increasing number of governments demand that an Electronic Medical Dossier (EMD) and, at a later stage, an Electronic Patient Dossier (EPD) need to be available to every party involved, organizations like the Dutch NICTIZ (www.nictiz.nl) work on standardizing information exchange between health care providers. An important emerging standard to exchange basic medical information is the HL7v3 standard. Apart from memory aids (see next paragraph) ICT solutions that inform people with dementia on their personal condition, appointments and care planning are still in the research and development stage.

4.3.2 Need for Support with Regard to Symptoms of Dementia

In the needs area support with regard to symptoms of dementia we included four websites and 20 publications.

4.3.2.1 ICT Compensation for Disabilities Such as Memory Problems

To help people with dementia undertake specific types of time-linked tasks (e.g. taking medication, keeping appointments or following a daily schedule) various possibilities of automatic reminders via Electronic Memory Aids (EMAs) are explored (e.g. Kim et al. 2000; Wilson et al. 2001; Hart et al. 2004). Kim et al. (2000) studied the use of a palmtop computer-based memory aid by persons with functional impairments of prospective memory and found this technology to be useful in a high proportion of patients for assisting memory-dependent functions. Hart et al. (2004) conducted a consumer survey study to ascertain experiences and attitudes regarding the use of portable electronic devices as memory and organizational aids. They concluded that these devices are acceptable or desirable for use as compensatory aids by consumers with moderate to severe brain injury. While these initiatives differ in approach, they agree on the usability of memory aids for persons with dementia, the importance of defining their own reminders and of giving them and their informal carers control over the reminders (e.g. Wilson et al. 2001; Inglis et al. 2003). Most researchers recognize the importance of involving informal carers in the implementation of EMAs as carers motivate the person with dementia to use the EMA but also benefit themselves, as use of an EMA by a person with dementia reduces feelings of worry in the informal carer (Szymkowiak et al. 2004).

Only a few studies have investigated the effect of EMAs for people with dementia (Van den Broek et al. 2000; Zanetti et al. 2000; Wilson et al. 2001.). Most studies are uncontrolled and based on a small sample, but justify hope for future development. Van den Broek et al. (2000) studied the use of the Voice Organizer, a device on which a message can be recorded by the user and that plays it back on a specified date and time. In the patients with memory problems that participated in the study the prospective memory improved directly after the device was taken into use.

Zanetti et al. (2000) asked five patients with Alzheimer's Disease to conduct seven prospective memory tasks on set times with the help of an electronic agenda and compared the effort with a control condition in which the same tasks had to be performed without the electronic agenda. All participants performed significantly better on the memory tasks when using the electronic agenda. Wilson et al. (2001) report on the effectiveness and usability of the "NeuroPage" system (Hersh and Treadgold 1994), a pager system which allows for a large number of reminders and prompts for various activities (www.neuropage.nhs.uk). Within a mixed diagnostic group with memory disorders, including people with dementia, NeuropPage as well as a pocket-computer memory enhancement system were evaluated and found to be workable although motivation and remembering to enter relevant information did limit overall usefulness (Wilson et al. 2001). EMAs appear particularly suited to support prospective memory and, although they are generally more expensive than non-electronic memory aids, require little training (see review Fritschy et al. 2004).

An electronic calendar to aid persons with memory problems or cognitive impairment, called the Forget-Me-Not device, was produced within the European Technology, Ethics and Dementia (TED) project and could be useful for persons who are confused about day and date (Holte et al. 1998). An EMA informing the person verbally, using vocal recordings, of specific appointments or tasks, also showed positive effects (Oriani et al. 2003). Inglis et al. (2003) and Szymkowiak et al. (2004) utilized a Personal Digital Assistant (PDA) to remind users of daily tasks, telephone numbers, appointments and birthdays. Users appreciated the device, though some visually or hearing impaired users preferred a reminder in the form of vibration.

Baruch et al. (2004) observed beneficial effects of computer systems on orientation, feelings of anxiety and independency in a patient suffering from Alzheimer's disease. Computer screens in the bedroom and living room reduced the needed support and the number of night time calls to the informal carer.

Within the multi-national ENABLE project (enabling technologies for people with dementia) 12 existing products (-concepts) were identified and their effectiveness to support memory, improve quality of life and reduce the carer burden was assessed. These assistive technologies were found to facilitate independent living and some devices may reduce anxiety in people with dementia as well as their informal carers (Gilliard and Hagen et al. 2004). EMAs, sometimes combined with interventions like visual imagery, errorless learning or spaced retrieval techniques, proved efficacious in stimulating memory in people with dementia (see review Grandmaison and Simard 2003).

Cognitive intervention is another approach to support people with dementia in their memory function and can be presented utilizing video conference, computer-based, or Internet-based systems.

In comparing cognitive intervention via a video conference system with face-to-face intervention, Poon et al. (2005) found telemedicine to be feasible, effective on memory, language and attention and highly accepted in people with dementia. Hofman et al. (1996) used an interactive computer-based program to train people with dementia to use a touch screen and showed improved performance in computer-program tasks. To determine the usefulness of an Interactive Multimedia Internet-based System (IMIS) in people with suspected Alzheimer's disease, Tárraga et al. (2006) compared IMIS in combination with an Integrated Psycho-stimulation Program (IPP) and pharmacological treatment to IPP combined with pharmacological treatment and pharmacological treatment alone. They found both IMIS and IPP to improve cognition and the IMIS program to provide improvement above that seen with IPP alone.

4.3.2.2 ICT Supporting the Carer, Flexibly and Personalized, in Instrumental Care

Formal and informal carers in a number of European and North-American countries utilize forms of telemedicine such as video conferencing, telemonitoring and telecare to create more capacity by reducing travel time and increase quality of care by allowing more frequent contact and quick referrals to a specialist. Several projects aimed to develop telecare home services that enable persons with dementia to live independently and offer support to their informal carers.

The European Fourth Framework Program (FP4) project ACTION (Assisting Carers using Telematics Interventions to meet Older persons Needs) focused on the empowerment of family carers to help maintain autonomy, independence and quality of life in frail elderly. Familiar electronic equipment like TV and telephone was combined with modern ICT to improve carers' coping skills in daily care and emergency interventions and to offer financial information and emotional support (Magnusson et al. 1998). A Swedish contribution to the project comprised a videophone to facilitate communication between health care providers and patients and their families. Magnusson et al. (2002) found that families were quicker to request information, education and support from professional carers and valued the informal support network of family carers to share experiences.

The FP5 project TeleCARE aimed to design and develop a flexible infrastructure of remote supervision and assistance services to facilitate independent lifestyles and to improve quality of life, confidence, well-being and safety in elderly people, including people with dementia. Partial validation was achieved with field assessments involving four classes of potential users including elderly and their relatives and health care providers. However, field tests for fine tuning and acceptance of the technology still need to be carried out (Camarinha-Matos and Asfaramesh 2004). Another telecare project is the "Tunstall telecare system", which can be tailored to suit the needs of people with dementia and protect them from dangers such as wandering, fires and floods (www.tunstalltown.com).

Within the "Safe-at-home" project, Woolham (2005) conducted a large-scale study into the effect of different items of assistive and telecare technology. An intervention group of 233 people with dementia was compared to a matched control group of 173. After intervention the two groups differed significantly in the number of services received, visits and contact hours per week, resulting in lower costs in the intervention group. The technology was found reliable and a majority of carers reported reduced feelings of concern for a person's safety. Almost half of the carers felt the project had improved the confidence of the user in their ability to look after themselves safely.

The experiences of 19 informal carers with a web-based home monitoring system, consisting of broadband Internet access, an Ethernet card, the Xanboo Smart Home Management system and a cell phone with text messaging, were explored by Kinney et al. (2004) in the SAFE house project. Carers received training on how to use the system prior to installation and were able to use the system during the intervention period of 24 weeks. Researchers reported reduced carer burden. Cell-phone alerts facilitated keeping track of loved ones and as relatives called more often, relationships improved (Kinney et al. 2004).

4.3.2.3 ICT Support for People with Dementia and Carers with Regard to Behavioural and Psychological Changes and How to Cope with Them

Information on behavioural and psychological changes in people with dementia, how to cope with them and where to find support can be found on websites of Alzheimer societies (e.g. www.alzheimer-nederland.nl). Alzheimer Nederland also offers a 24-h telephone service for information, support and advice. The Dutch site www.hulpgids.nl offers psychiatric consultation, forum discussions and fellow-patient contact. On www.vraagwijzer.nl one can get help clarifying a health care demand, get advice on adequate care and support in how to receive the desired type of care.

The Geriatric Research, Education and Clinical Centre (GRECC) of the Minneapolis Department of Veteran Affairs Medical Centre offers practical online information on a number of topics related to caring for a patient with dementia (e.g. how to handle a loved one's decline, how to cope with bowel and urinary incontinence) (http://james.psych.umn.edu/~grecc/caring.htm; Long and Williams 2005). The US website www.alzonline.net provides Internet- and telephone-based support and education for people with Alzheimer's disease and other dementias as well as support for their carers. Utilizing training videos and downloadable information, the site offers classes to address a wide range of topics related to dementia care (e.g. medication management, dealing with the stress of caring and performing daily tasks). An initial program evaluation showed reasonable effectiveness of AlzOnline's Positive Caregiving Classes. Carer self-efficacy improved and subjective carer burden was reduced but positive dimensions of the care giving experience and perceptions of time burden in providing care were unaltered (Glueckauf et al.

2004). The efficacy of "Care-giver's Friend", an Internet-based multimedia support program designed to support family carers employed in the workforce, was tested by Beauchamp et al. (2005) in 299 participants using a pre-test/post-test design. Results showed significant benefits on carer depression and anxiety and improvements in perceived stress, strain and positive aspects of care giving.

Guiding the behaviour (e.g. to go to a day care centre, eat more meals) of people with dementia by music and sung messages output by an IC recorder was found to be highly effective (Yasuda et al. 2006). The researchers suggest that music can have a strong effect on mental stability and the method can easily be applied to other activities of daily life.

4.3.2.4 Emotional Support for People with Dementia and Carers

White and Dorman (2000) analysed the contents of messages posted on an Alzheimer mail group and concluded that the opportunity to share, unburden or vent, is perceived as empowering and helpful to carers. Almost every Alzheimer association offers a website where people with dementia and their carers can join forums, post messages or chat with fellow sufferers (e.g. http://www.alzheimer-nederland.nl, http://www.pick.nl). Many Alzheimer associations also have a 24-h telephone support service for emotional support and information on regional support services like Alzheimer café's and meeting centres.

An Internet-based application called Alzheimer's Carer Internet Support System (ACISS), designed to provide carers with clinical, decision-making and emotional support, was evaluated in a 6-month field trial of 42 carer/patient dyads. Preliminary results showed the system to be beneficial to carers of people with dementia (Vehvilainen et al. 2002).

4.3.3 Need for Social Contact and Company for the Person with Dementia

In the need area for social contact and company 11 publications were included. Simplified mobile phones for elderly persons to contact informal carers or relatives directly have recently been developed. Lekeu et al. (2002) demonstrated that people with mild dementia are able to learn how to use a mobile phone with an "errorless learning" method (Clare et al. 2000). The "Mobile Telecoach", a one-button mobile phone which allows direct answering, had an effect on positive social experiences and self-esteem in people with dementia. However, users were not satisfied with its size, weight and battery life (Kort 2005). The FP4 project MORE was aimed at redesigning existing mobile phones and simplifying the user interface to meet the many differing needs of elderly and disabled people. Various MORE-based telephones with an integral GPS function were produced by Benefon, but none of these have come into use as navigation support for people with disabilities (Lindström 2005).

Within the FP4 project TASC (Telematic Applications Supporting Cognition), five software modules were developed for supporting persons with developmental disability, brain injury or dementia in information provision, communication, environmental control, planning and time management. The TASC system runs on a standard computer; the modules can be used separately or together, are designed to be compatible with future extensions and can be programmed to fit the needs of an individual user. Usability and functional effectiveness of alpha-versions of the system were trialled with representatives of user groups. The amended system was implemented with 18 users across five validation sites. The field trials indicate that the TASC system can reduce the need for help from others with daily activities, leading to increased independence and quality of life and reduced costs for assistance and institutional care (Ager and Aalykke 2001). The ENABLE project included a number of devices to provide pleasure or comfort and facilitate communication such as a picture gramophone (a do-it-yourself multimedia program), a "My history" device (PC with touch screen showing pictures of people and places with familiar voice narrative) and a pre-programmable telephone (calls initiated by just pressing one large button containing a name or photo). Trials among people with mild to moderate dementia indicate that these assistive technologies can enhance well-being by giving positive experiences and reduce anxiety in people with dementia and their informal carers (Gilliard and Hagen 2004).

The "Musical Memory Lane" built in a 1930s Philco radio cabinet and the "Video Memory Lane" housed in a 1950s television cabinet present nostalgic music and videos to people with Alzheimer's Disease in an easy-to-access, push-button, picture format. Systematic observations indicate that the Memory Lanes have a favourable impact on engagement, stimulate positive affect and activity-related talking, while also reducing fidgeting (Olsen et al. 2000).

"Televisits", contact between elderly people living in a nursing home and their family via a videophone, was demonstrated to promote social contact by Mickus and Luz (2002). In a similar study, Sävenstedt et al. (2003) showed that a videophone as a means of communication between patient and family reduced feelings of guilt in family members, allowed more frequent visits than was possible with face-to-face visits and let family members see the physical and emotional state of the patient on a daily basis. In some cases the conversations were more focused and of better quality than during face-to-face visits. In most cases, however, more emphasis was placed on the family member to direct and lead the conversations which was seen by many as demanding. The relationship between staff and family members improved as a side effect of staff helping the patient use the videophone.

Tamura et al. (2004) found that a motorized toy dog can effectively reduce wandering and agitation after dinner in people with dementia. The robot dog AIBO as well as a motorized toy dog proved to be effective in increasing patient activity and spontaneous speech during occupational therapy. Sakairi (2004) showed that the introduction of AIBO increased the number of utterances in people with dementia. These results indicate that socialization and social activity can increase in the presence of a toy dog and AIBO. Alm et al. (2003) suggest that with the use of multimedia as a source of reminiscence, patients exhibit more control of the direction of the conversation. They developed a touch screen display to convey photographs, video or music and compared it to traditional reminiscence methods. The patients using the multimedia system showed stronger and more prolonged engagement during the conversations.

4.3.4 Need for Health Monitoring and Perceived Safety

Implementing monitoring technologies and detection devices or alarm systems inside and outside the home of elderly persons is potentially useful to enhance (perceived) safety and security of the person suffering from dementia as well as carers. Over the last few decades, detection devices and alarm systems for health problems and safety have been developed for different diagnostic groups, but we found only 12 studies that investigated the effect of these devices among people with dementia.

In a study comparing four biomechanical activity devices to index wandering, Algase et al. (2003) found the stepwatch particularly able to assess amount and daily course of wandering behaviour in people with dementia. In this context, Boundary alarms (activated by a wristband) or electronic tagging with bracelets and monitoring stations were found to be effective, reliable and successful in detecting wandering as well as reducing patient and carer stress (Blackburn 1988; Miskelly 2004). A bedside monitoring system tested in a hospital setting with three patients with dementia who frequently wandered during the night, additionally provides floor lighting upon wandering detection and relays an alarm to a personal handheld device alerting the carer to the situation so that the necessary intervention can be performed (Masuda et al. 2002). A straying prevention system developed by Lin et al. (2006) can counteract wandering without interfering with the daily life activities of the person suffering from dementia. The system consists of indoor residence monitoring, outdoor activity monitoring, emergency rescue service and remote monitoring that can be accessed via a number of mobile devices such as a mobile phone, PDA, notebook or computer. The indoor monitor detects movement between certain areas within the home. Outdoor activities, accompanied or unaccompanied, are monitored in a pre-set activity area, which is activated by pressing a button on the location tracking device. Messages or alarms, respectively, are generated and forwarded via mobile communication (GSM) if the patient leaves the home environment or the activity area. In case of an emergency, the person with dementia can activate an emergency button which sends a message to the call centre where the situation, location and geographical information and location coordinates are analyzed and relayed to care providers, search teams and family members. Conversely, through the secure remote monitoring facility included in the system, family members or care providers can access patient's location information at any time by logging onto the system. Although it was not tested with patients of the target group, the system was expected to be beneficial in helping locate elderly people with dementia by 11 volunteers who reviewed the system. Paavilainen et al. (2005) tested an active social alarm system, IST Vivago® WristCare, which provides continuous telemetric monitoring of the user's activity. Results of this study support the use of telemetric actigraphy in long-term screening and follow-up of elderly subjects for sleep and circadian rhythm-related problems associated with dementia and changes in functional capacity.

A fully automatic multi-sensor system composed of Infra Red (IR) sensors connected to a personal computer installed in a patient's room was evaluated by Chan et al. (2002). This smart tool system proved valid in assessing and recording data on activities such as getting out of bed, mobility and travel patterns of a psychotic patient with moderate cognitive decline and behavioural disorders.

Global Positioning Systems (GPS) can also assist in locating people with dementia. Recently, Miskelly (2005) tested a mobile phone with GPS to help families of dementia sufferers if their relative happens to wander off. The person with dementia carries the mobile phone when leaving the house. If a carer or relative needs to know his or her whereabouts, a 24-h control centre can be called. By getting the coordinates of the phone they can pinpoint the person's location with an accuracy of 5 m, enabling help to be sent quickly.

The suitability of GPS systems for location tracking is highlighted by Shimizu et al. (2000) who developed a system that locates the wandering individual to a range of 100–200 m. The system was tested in various conditions such as adverse weather and close proximity of tall buildings. Results showed that despite these adverse conditions, the location accuracy and frequency were sufficient for application in dementia wandering.

The Personal Handy-phone System, worn by the patient as a pendant, could transmit the patient's position with an accuracy of 60 m to a personal computer. The computer generates a map of the area, and then automatically sends this map via email to the carer who can view it on a mobile phone (Ogawa et al. 2004).

Applying a user-driven design approach Orpwood et al. (2005) developed and evaluated a smart home environment consisting of different services that aimed to assist people with dementia in various areas. During the night, for example, a lighting system was activated if a patient had left the bed. On returning to bed the lights would fade off after a few minutes. However, failure to return to bed after a pre-defined period of time would result in the communication system telling the patient that it is night time and they should go to bed. Furthermore, the system communicated to the patients when they approached an exit during the night and verbally reminded the patient to return to bed. Next to night monitoring, the system incorporated a cooking monitor service, detecting problems and potential dangers during the cooking process. During evaluations the cooker monitor worked well. However, it caused some irritation to users when the cooker was turned off under false positive situations.

The "eHealth Strategic Objective" of the Information Society Technologies research program of the European Commission is aiming to create an "intelligent environment" that allows ubiquitous management of each person's health status, assisting patients and health professionals in coping with major health challenges. The focus is on key technologies, such as biosensors and secure communications in "smart clothes" and implants, as well as software tools for monitoring and managing health status and patient safety. As far as we know such technologies are not yet being applied and validated for persons with dementia.

4.4 Conclusion and Discussion

The aim of this review was to get an overview of ICT solutions that successfully supports people with dementia in the areas of obtaining generalized and personal information, coping with symptoms of dementia, maintaining social contact and company and enhancing (feelings of) safety.

4.4.1 Available ICT-Based Services per Needs Area

Based on this literature study we can conclude that digital *information* on dementia, health companies, services and support offerings or financial and legal issues is provided with varying quality on multiple websites, as well as by digital social charts. A majority of these sites offer useful tips and support for carers but seem less attuned to the person suffering from dementia. This applies to the web design as well as to the information offered. Unfortunately, we did not find research in which the websites were tested on helpfulness for the target group. Additionally, an overriding drawback of all digital information is its generic nature. Demand-orientated, personalized information is still difficult to obtain. As the need for personalized and context-sensitive information clearly exists (van der Roest et al. 2007; van der Roest et al. 2009), future development of digital information systems should take these aspects into account.

In the last decade various ICT solutions were developed to support people with dementia and their carers in their everyday problems that arise from the *symptoms* associated with dementia. External memory aids in the form of reminders (to take medication or keep appointments) or cognitive interventions with Internet-based multimedia systems, including familiar equipment such as TV or PC, have proven efficacious in stimulating memory as well as enhancing feelings of independence and autonomy in the person with dementia. Several devices were developed to compensate for cognitive disabilities in the ENABLE project (e.g. a cooker usage monitor). All in all, these studies show that persons with dementia are not only capable of handling electronic equipment, but also benefit in terms of more confidence and enhanced positive affect, thereby indirectly reducing the carer's perceived burden. Information and emotional support for carers in coping with dementia symptoms furthermore is available through web forums and chat rooms, video-training and telephone services. Though web-based interventions seem promising especially to help meeting the various needs of people with dementia and carers in an effective and less time-consuming way, instrumental ICT support for coping with behavioural and psychological changes in dementia is, however, relatively disregarded as yet. People with dementia and their carers have access to online information (e.g. site of the Alzheimer Association), support (e.g. "Carer's Friend"; Beauchamp et al. 2005), education (e.g. AlzOnline's Positive Care giving classes; Glueckauf et al. 2004) and advice (e.g. online consultation of psychiatrist on www.hulpgids.nl) on coping with behavioural and psychological changes. However, apart from a study in which recorded music in combination with sung messages was found to be highly effective in guiding the behaviour of people with dementia (Yasuda et al. 2006), no proven successful instrumental ICT solutions for coping with behavioural and psychological changes were found. The integration of different technologies into a combined modular system, as piloted in several European projects such as FP4-TASC and FP5-TeleCARE, looks promising. Patients not only made less use of conventional health services, but also reported less negative feelings. Further effort into integrating different systems into a service bundle delivered to patients is therefore recommended.

Support for *social contact and company* is realized through simplified mobile phones or videophones, that have been reported to facilitate communication between people with dementia and their family or friends. Enhanced positive affect as well as increased activity and communication levels have been observed with computer software providing music or video memories or robotics, such as a toy dog or an entertainment robot. These technical solutions proved to be easily implemented and of great benefit to the person with dementia and their carers.

Finally, we found several ICT solutions for *health monitoring and to enhance perceived safety*. GPS technology for tracking wandering or lost persons as well as monitoring systems to detect fire or gas leakage or signal night-time activity allow for unobtrusive yet efficient assessments of safety. Additionally, people with dementia and their carers report enhanced feelings of safety and security and less fear and anxiety. Dissemination and implementation of these systems into households are therefore advisable. The monitoring of biological functions in people with dementia is still in its infancy. Unobtrusive, ubiquitous monitoring and management of a person's health using an "intelligent environment" (e.g. the "eHealth Strategic Objective") seems to have potential for the future but has yet to prove its efficacy in the field.

4.4.2 Limitations of the Current Study

In order to make the review study practical a number of limitations are present both in the searching process and the analysis. A first restriction concerned the focus of the study. Only ICT solutions that could contribute to meet the most frequently mentioned *unmet* needs by people with dementia and their informal carers (see Table 4.1) were included in the study. ICT solutions in other needs areas were therefore not included in this study.

A second restriction limited the searching process to a number of databases which covered both the clinical and technical aspects of the study. The databases PubMed, PsychInfo, Cinahl, INSPEC, IEEE and Google (Scholar) were used in the searching process with a total of 165 articles found. Although this selection may have caused us to miss relevant articles, we feel the variety of articles found provides a good overview of the state of the art of ICT solutions for the selected needs of people with dementia.

A third restriction was that we included only articles that reported on ICT solutions that were proven to be helpful for people with dementia and/or their carers and that were published before 15th November 2006. ICT solutions that are currently on the market and potentially useful for the target group, but for which no publications were found on the usefulness for people with dementia and/or their carers, are therefore not included in this review.

4.4.3 Societal Relevance

ICT support for needs that are unmet by the present care and welfare services could optimize the care for people with dementia and their carers and thus enhances their quality of life.

Whether people with dementia or their informal carers actually make use of and benefit from available ICT applications and services will partly depend on the attitude of health care professionals towards these solutions (e.g. Larner 2003). People with dementia and their informal carers are most likely to learn about available ICT solutions through their general practitioner, specialist, insurance company or care and welfare organizations. In order to inform their clients well, health care professionals should be aware of current and new ICT developments and services. This review gives an overview of successfully and partially successfully applied ICT solutions for people with dementia and their carers and therefore can help health care professionals to get informed on this subject and transfer this knowledge to their clients.

Not all ICT applications and services on today's market have been tested in advance or applied successfully for people with dementia. Although some untested systems could be beneficial to people with dementia or their carers, one cannot be sure of the efficacy of these systems. Only when the system is installed and in use, will the actual effect become clear, in the worst case causing financial, administrative or emotional difficulties for the end-user. Without pretending to be complete, this review tried to focus specifically on ICT solutions that have been successfully tested on people with dementia or their informal carers and have proven to be helpful. This review can therefore support professionals, people with dementia and their informal carers in selecting a specific solution. The information gathered in this review can also be used by health care professionals, policy makers and account managers of insurance companies to assess whether an application or service should be included in National Health Service packages or should be subsidized from health care funds.

As people with mild to moderate dementia seem capable of expressing their needs and do so from a different perspective than their informal carer (Dröes et al. 2006; van der Roest et al. 2007), ICT solutions should be developed in dialogue with the target users. Feedback from people with dementia and their carers during the development process can be used to make the final product better attuned to their needs, more personalized and more helpful (COGKNOW Consortium 2006; Sixsmith et al. 2007).

4.4.4 Technological Interest and Research Recommendations

Previous research on ICT solutions that aims to meet the unmet needs of people with dementia and their carers in the need areas we focused on in this review study primarily focused on two areas. Most studies concerned general information on the disease; how to cope with the consequences and service offerings on the one hand, and on the safety and monitoring of the person with dementia in various situations on the other hand. The majority of the latter solutions were particularly concerned with stray prevention and adopted a number of varying techniques to detect or locate the person with dementia when wandering both within and outside of the home environment. In the majority of solutions for stray prevention and detection, a warning system was adopted to alert carers or close family members to particular situations that could pose a risk to the person with dementia. Another area that the research explored was that of social contact and providing a basis for allowing a person with dementia to communicate better with others. The research articles found in this area highlighted the need for technology to allow persons with dementia to improve on their communication skills with others. Two studies showed that by using videophone technology, the quantity and quality of conversations between the person with dementia and others would be enhanced (Mickus and Luz 2002; Savenstedt et al. 2003).

One area that was relatively poorly represented was support for persons with dementia to compensate for their disabilities. Although quite a number of solutions were found for memory problems that could potentially be applicable to person with dementia, for some there was no direct evidence that they were effective in the target group. Therefore, these systems were excluded from the review. In a similar fashion there were a number of systems that aimed to provide help with daily living activities such as brushing your teeth; however, these solutions were never tested on people with dementia and were therefore also excluded from the review. Though successfully applied in a single study (Yasuda et al. 2006), instrumental ICT support for coping with behavioural and psychological symptoms in dementia is relatively disregarded as yet and the same holds for personalized information on the diagnosis, condition and personal care appointments. In summary it can be noted that there is a lack of ICT research conducted for two of the four areas that this review process addresses, namely support for obtaining personalized information and instrumental support for dealing with symptoms of dementia, such as memory problems, behavioural and psychological changes and problems with daily activities.

It is recommended that future studies should concentrate on integrating and applying current techniques and solutions in real-life situations with persons with dementia. This research and development process should be user-driven "to ensure that devices and systems are grounded within a thorough understanding of the needs, preferences and desires of potential users" (Sixsmith et al. 2007). Special attention should be given to ICT solutions that provide personalized information; compensate for disabilities such as memory problems; help people with dementia and their carers to cope with the behavioural and psychological changes associated with the dementia; and provide help with daily activities, including pleasant activities (Dröes et al. 2006; Sixsmith et al. 2007). The former two need particular attention in producing new ideas on how technology can be of assistance for the target group. An example of a personalized information service is the dynamic interactive social chart for dementia care (DEM-DISC) that provides people with dementia and their informal and formal carers with tailor-made information on regional and national care and support services (and service bundles) (Dröes et al. 2005a, b). ICT solutions for helping people to cope with behavioural and psychological changes and help with daily activities require selection of existing smart home solutions and the subsequent adaptation and testing of them for persons with dementia. All of the authors of this review participate or are indirectly involved in the COGKNOW project (2006) that aims at helping people with mild dementia navigate through their day. The project focuses on developing integrated ICT solutions for frequently mentioned unmet needs by people with dementia and their carers (Dröes et al. 2006; van der Roest et al. 2007), including memory support, support for social contact and daily activities and support for enhancing feelings of safety.

The majority of the studies found included small user groups and were uncontrolled, which makes it hard to generalize their outcomes. Therefore, a second recommendation would be to test the effectiveness of ICT solutions on a larger scale in, preferably, randomized controlled trials before implementing them in the care for people with dementia.

Acknowledgements The study was conducted within the framework of two projects: the FReeband User eXperience (FRUX) project that was financed by the Dutch Ministry of Economic Affairs under contract BSIK 03025, Dioraphte Foundation, RCOAK, NHDI, Foundation het Zonnehuis and the Alzheimer and Neuropsychiatrie Foundation and the COGKNOW project that is funded by the European Commission's Information Society Technologies (IST) program under grant 034025.

References

Ager, A., Aalykke, S. (2001) TASC: A microcomputer support system for persons with cognitive disabilities. British Journal of Educational Technology, 32:373–377.

Algase, D.L., Beattie, E.R.A., Leitsch, S.A., Beel-Bates, C.A. (2003) Biomechanical activity devices to index wandering behaviour in dementia. American Journal of Alzheimer's Disease and Other Dementias, 18:85–92.

Alm, N., Dye, R., Gowans, G., Campbell, J., Astell, A., Ellis, M. (2003). Designing an interface usable by people with dementia. ACM SIGCAPH Computers and the Physically Handicapped, June–September, pp. 156–157.

Baruch, J., Downs, M., Baldwin, C., Bruce, E. (2004). A case study in the use of technology to reassure and support a person with dementia. In: J. Moriarty (ed.) Innovative Practice, Dementia: The International Journal of Social Research and Practice, 3(3):371–392.

Beauchamp, N., Irvine, A.B., Seeley, J., Johnson, B. (2005) Worksite-based internet multimedia program for family caregivers of persons with dementia. Gerontologist, 45:793–801.

Biegel, D.E., Bass, D.M., Schulz, R., Morycz, R. (1993) Predictors of in-home and out-of-home service use by family caregivers of Alzheimer's disease patients. Journal of Aging and Health, 5:419–438.

Blackburn, P. (1988) Freedom to wander. Nursing Times, 84:54–55.

Brodaty, H., Thomson, C., Thompson, C., Fine, M. (2005) Why caregivers of people with dementia and memory loss don't use services. International Journal of Geriatric Psychiatry, 20:537–546.

Broek, M.D.V.D., Downes, J., Johnson, Z., Dayus, B., Hilton, N. (2000) Evaluation of an electronic memory aid in the neuropsychological rehabilitation of prospective memory deficits. Brain Injury, 14:455–462.

Burns, A. (2000) The burden of Alzheimer's disease. The International Journal of Neuropsychopharmacology, 3:31–38.

Camarinha-Matos, L., Asfaramesh, H. (2004) TeleCARE: Collaborative virtual elderly care support communities. Journal on Information Technology in Healthcare, 2:73–86.

Chan, M., Campo, E., Laval, E., Estève, D. (2002) Validation of a remote monitoring system for the elderly: Application to mobility measurements. Technology and Health Care, 10:391–399.

Clare, L., Wilson, B.A., Carter, G., Breen, K., Gosses, A., Hodges, J.R. (2000) Intervening with everyday memory problems in dementia of Alzheimer type: An errorless learning approach. Journal of Clinical and Experimental Neuropsychology, 22:132–146.

Clare, L. (2002) We'll fight it as long as we can: coping with the onset of Alzheimer's disease. Aging and Mental Health, 6:139–148.

Coe, M., Neufeld, A. (1999) Male caregivers' use of formal support. Western Journal of Nursing Research, 21:568–588.

COGKNOW Consortium. (2006). COGKNOW: Helping people with dementia navigate their day. Description of Work, Project Proposal, EU Contract no. 034025.

Cox, C. (1997) Findings from a state-wide program of respite care: A comparison of service users, stoppers, and nonusers. Gerontologist, 37:511–517.

Cummings, J.L., Mega, M., Gray, K., Rosenberg-Thompson, S., Carusi, D.A., Gornbein, J. (1994) The neuropsychiatric inventory: Comprehensive assessment of psychopathology in dementia. Neurology, 44:2308–2314.

Dröes, R.M., Lindeman, E.M., Breebaart, E., van Tilburg, W. (1996). Determinanten van belasting van verzorgers van mensen die lijden aan dementie. In: R.M. Dröes (ed.) Amsterdamse Ontmoetingscentra; een nieuwe vorm van ondersteuning voor mensen met dementie en hun verzorgers. Eindrapport 1996. Thesis Publishers, Amsterdam, pp. 89–118.

Dröes, R.M., van Hout, H.P.J., van der Ploeg, E.S. (2004). Camberwell Assessment of Need for the Elderly (CANE). Revised version IV. Nederlandse Vertaling. VU Medisch Centrum, Amsterdam.

Dröes, R.M., Meiland, F.J.M., Doruff, C., Varodi, I., Akkermans, H., Baida, Z., Faber, E., Haaker, T., Moelaert, F., Kartseva, V., Tan, Y.H. (2005a) A dynamic interactive social chart in dementia care. Attuning demand and supply in the care for persons with dementia and their carers. In: L. Bos, S. Laxminarayan, A. Marsh (eds.) Medical and Care Compunetics, Studies in Health Technology and Informatics. IOS Press, The Netherlands, England, 2(114):210–220.

Dröes, R.M., Meiland, F.J.M., van der Roest, H.G., Maroccini, R., Slagter, R.S., Baida, Z., Haaker, T., Kartseva, V., Hulstijn, J., Schmieman, R., Akkermans, H., Faber, E., Tan, Y.H. (2005b). Opportunities for we-centric service bundling in dementia care. Freeband FRUX Project, Amsterdam.

Dröes, R.M., Boelens, E.J., Bos, J., Meihuizen, L., Ettema, T.P., Gerritsen, D.L., Hoogeveen, F., de Lange, J., Schölzel-Dorenbos, C. (2006) Quality of life in dementia in perspective; an explorative study of variations in opinions among people with dementia and their professional caregivers, and in literature. Dementia: The International Journal of Social Research and Practice, 5:533–558.

Duijnstee, M. (1992). De belasting van familieleden van dementerenden. Intro, Nijkerk.

Dunkin, J.J., Anderson-Hanley, C. (1998) Dementia caregiver burden: a review of the literature and guidelines for assessment and intervention. Neurology, 51:S53–S60.

Ferri, C.P., Prince, M., Brayne, C., Brodaty, H., Fratiglioni, L., Ganguli, M., Hall, K., Hasegawa, K., Hendrie, H., Huang, Y., Jorm, A., Mathers, C., Menezes, P.R., Rimmer, E., Scazufca, M. (2005) Global prevalence of dementia: A Delphi consensus study. Lancet, 366:2112–2117.

Freeman, E., Clare, L., Savitch, N., Royan, L., Litherland, R., Lindsay, M. (2005) Improving website accessibility for people with early stage dementia: A preliminary investigation. Aging and Mental Health, 9:442–448.

Fritschy, E.P., Kessels, R.P., Postma, A. (2004) External memory aids for patients with dementia: A literature study on efficacy and applicability. Tijdschr Gerontol Geriatr, 35:234–239.

Gilliard, J., Hagen, I. (2004). Enabling technologies for people with dementia. Cross-National Analysis Report, D4.4.1. QLK6-CT-2000-00653, pp. 1–69.

Glueckauf, R.L., Ketterson, T.U., Loomis, J.S., Dages, P. (2004) Online support and education for dementia caregivers: Overview, utilization, and initial program evaluation. Telemedicine Journal and e-Health, 10:223–232.

Grandmaison, E., Simard, M. (2003) A critical review of memory stimulation programs in Alzheimer's disease. Journal of Neuropsychiatry and Clinical Neurosciences, 15:130–144.

Gwyther, L.P. (1998) Social issues of the Alzheimer's patient and family. American Journal of Medicine, 104:17S–21S.

Hancock, G.A., Woods, B., Challis, D., Orrell, M. (2006) The needs of older people with dementia in residential care. International Journal of Geriatric Psychiatry, 21:43–49.

Hart, T., Buchhofer, R., Vaccaro, M. (2004) Portable electronic devices as memory and organizational aids after traumatic brain injury: A consumer survey study. Journal of Head Trauma Rehabilitation, 19:351–365.

Hassol, A., Walker, J.M., Kidder, D., Rokita, K., Young, D., Pierdon, S., Deitz, D., Kuck, S., Ortiz, E. (2004) Patient experiences and attitudes about access to a patient electronic health care record and linked web messaging. Journal of the American Medical Informatics Association, 11:505–513.

Health Council of the Netherlands. (2002/04) Dementia. The Hague, Health Council of the Netherlands.

Hersh, N.A., Treadgold, L.G. (1994) NeuroPage: The rehabilitation of memory dysfunction by prosthetic memory and cueing. Neurorehabilitation, 4:187–197.

Hofmann, M., Hock, C., Kuhler, A., Muller-Spahn, F. (1996) Interactive computer-based cognitive training in patients with Alzheimer's disease. Journal of Psychiatric Research, 30:493–501.

Holte, T., Hagen, I., Björneby, S. (1998). Evaluation of an electronic calendar as helping aid for persons suffering from memory problems or cognitive impairment. Report of the TED-Group.

Honeyman, A., Cox, B., Fisher, B. (2005) Potential impacts of patient access to their electronic care records. Information for Primary Care, 13:55–60.

Inglis, E.A., Szymkowiak, A., Gregor, P., Newell, A.F., Hine, N., Shah, P., Wilson, B.A., Evans, J. (2003) Issues surrounding the user-centred development of a new interactive memory aid. Universal Access in the Information Society, 2:226–234.

Kim, H.J., Burke, D.T., Dowds, M.M., Jr., Boone, K.A., Park, G.J. (2000) Electronic memory aids for outpatient brain injury: Follow-up findings. Brain Injury, 14:187–196.

Kinney, J., Kart, C.S., Murdoch, L., Conley, C. (2004) Striving to provide safety assistance for families of elders: The SAFE House project. Dementia: The International Journal of Social Research and Practice, 3:351–370.

Koffman, J., Taylor, S. (1997) The needs of caregivers. Elder Care, 9:16–19.

Kort, S. (2005). Mobile coaching. A pilot study into the user-friendliness and effects of Mobile Coaching on the wellbeing of people with dementia and their informal caregivers. Faculty of Psychology, Vrije Universiteit, Amsterdam.

Larner, A.J. (2003) Use of the internet and of the NHS direct telephone helpline for medical information by a cognitive function clinic population. International Journal of Geriatric Psychiatry, 18:118–122.

Lauriks, S., Reinersmann, A., van der Roest, H., Meiland, F.J.M., Davies, R.J., Moelaert, F., Mulvenna, M.D., Nugent, C.D., Dröes, R.M. (2007 October) Review of ICT-based services for identified unmet needs in people with dementia. Ageing Research Reviews, 6(3):223–246.

Lekeu, F., Wojtasik, V., van der Linden, M., Salmon, E. (2002) Training early Alzheimer patients to use a mobile phone. Acta Neurologica Belgium, 102:114–121.

Lin, C.C., Chiu, M.J., Hsiao, C.C., Lee, R.G., Tsai, Y.S. (2006) Wireless health care service system for elderly with dementia. IEEE Transactions on Information Technology Biomedicine, 10:696–704.

Lindström, J.I. (2005) Navigation, alarming and positioning. A preliminary study conducted in Sweden by the Royal Institute of Technology (KTH), Department of Speech, Music and Hearing, on the Assignment of the National Post and Telecom agency (PTS). PTS-ER–2006–16.

Long, C.O., Williams, J.K. (2005) Exploring Alzheimer's disease on the Web. Nursing, 35:30–31.

Magnusson, L., Berthold, H., Chambers, M., Brito, L., Emery, D., Daly, T. (1998) Using telematics with older people: the ACTION project. Assisting carers using telematics interventions to meet older persons' needs. Nursing Standard, 13:36–40.

Magnusson, L., Hanson, E., Brito, L., Berthold, H., Chambers, M., Daly, T. (2002) Supporting family carers through the use of information and communication technology – the EU project ACTION. International Journal of Nursing Studies, 39:369–381.

Masuda, Y., Yoshimura, T., Nakajima, K., Nambu, M., Hayakawa, T., Tamura, T. (2002) Unconstrained monitoring of prevention of wandering the elderly. In: Engineering in Medicine and Biology, 24th Annual Conference and the Annual Fall Meeting of the Biomedical Engineering Society (EMBS/BMES Conference). Proceedings of the Second Joint, 2:1906–1907.

Mickus, M.A., Luz, C.C. (2002) Televisits: Sustaining long distance family relationships among institutionalized elders through technology. Aging Mental and Health, 6:387–396.

Miskelly, F. (2004) A novel system of electronic tagging in patients with dementia and wandering. Age and Ageing, 33:304–306.

Miskelly, F. (2005) Electronic tracking of patients with dementia and wandering using mobile phone technology. Age and Ageing, 34:497–499.

Ogawa, H., Yonezawa, Y., Maki, H., Sato, H., Caldwell, W.M. (2004). A mobile phone-based safety support system for wandering elderly persons. In: 26th Annual International Conference of the Engineering in Medicine and Biology Society (EMBC). Conference Proceedings 2: 3316–3317.

Olsen, R.V., Hutchings, B.L., Ehrenkrantz, E. (2000) "Media Memory Lane" interventions in an Alzheimer's day care centre. American Journal of Alzheimer's Disease and Other Dementias, 15:163–175.

Oriani, M., Moniz-Cook, E., Binetti, G., Zanieri, G., Frisoni, G.B., Geroldi, C., de Vreese, L.P., Zanetti, O. (2003) An electronic memory aid to support prospective memory in patients in the early stages of Alzheimer's disease: A pilot study. Aging and Mental Health, 7: 22–27.

Orpwood, R., Gibbs, C., Adlam, T., Faulkner, R., Meegahawatte, D. (2005) The design of smart homes for people with dementia – user-interface aspects. Universal Access in the Information Society, 4:156–164.

Paavilainen, P., Korhonen, I., Lotjonen, J., Cluitmans, L., Jylha, M., Sarela, A., Partinen, M. (2005) Circadian activity rhythm in demented and non-demented nursing-home residents measured by telemetric actigraphy. Journal of Sleep Research, 14:61–68.

Perry, J., Bontinen, K. (2001) Evaluation of a weekend respite program for persons with Alzheimer disease. Canadian Journal of Nursing Research, 33:81–95.

Poon, P., Hui, E., Dai, D., Kwok, T., Woo, J. (2005) Cognitive intervention for community-dwelling older persons with memory problems: Telemedicine versus face-to-face treatment. International Journal of Geriatric Psychiatry, 20:285–286.

Proctor, R., Testad, I. (2005) Carer stress-overview. In: A. Burns (ed.) Standards in Dementia Care. European Dementia Consensus Network Edcon. Taylor & Francis Group, New York, pp. 241–273.

Sakairi, K. (2004) Research of robot-assisted activity for the elderly with senile dementia in a group home. SICE 2004 Annual Conference, 3:2092–2094.

Savenstedt, S., Brulin, C., Sandman, P.O. (2003) Family members' narrated experiences of communicating via video-phone with patients with dementia staying at a nursing home. Journal of Telemedicine and Telecare, 9:216–220.

Shimizu, K., Kawamura, K., Yamamoto, K. (2000). Location system for dementia wandering. In: 22nd Annual International Conference of the IEEE Engineering in Medicine and Biology Society. Proceedings of the 22nd Annual International Conference of the IEEE, 2:1556–1559.

Sixsmith, A.J., Gibson, R.D., Orpwood, R.D., Torrington, J.M. (2007) Developing a technology 'wish-list' to enhance the quality of life of people with dementia. Gerontechnology, 6:2–19.

Szymkowiak, A., Morrison, K., Shah, P., Gregor, P., Evans, J., Newell, A.F., Wilson, B.A., Shofield, S. (2004). Memojog – an interactive memory aid with remote communication. In: S. Keates, J. Clarkson, P. Langdon, P. Robinson (eds.) Designing a More Inclusive World. Proceedings of 2nd Cambridge Workshop on Universal Access and Assistive Technology (CWUAAT) 22 April 2004, Cambridge, UK, pp. 15–24.

Tamura, T., Yonemitsu, S., Itoh, A., Oikawa, D., Kawakami, A., Higashi, Y., Fujimooto, T., Nakajima, K. (2004) Is an entertainment robot useful in the care of elderly people with severe dementia? Journal of Gerontology Series A: Biological Science and Medical Science, 59:83–85.

Tarraga, L., Boada, M., Modinos, G., Espinosa, A., Diego, S., Morera, A., Guitart, M., Balcells, J., Lopez, O.L., Becker, J.T. (2006) A randomised pilot study to assess the efficacy of an interactive, multimedia tool of cognitive stimulation in Alzheimer's disease. Journal of Neurology, Neurosurgery and Psychiatry, 77:1116–1121.

van der Roest, H.G., Meiland, F.J.M., Maroccini, R., Comijs, H.C., Jonker, C., Dröes, R.M. (June, 2007) Subjective needs of people with dementia: A review of the literature. International Psychogeriatric, 19(3):559–592.

Van der Roest, H.G., Meiland, F.J.M., Comijs, H.C., Jansen, A.P., van Hout, H.P.J. (2009). What do community-dwelling people with dementia need? A survey among those who are known to care and welfare services. International Psychogeriatrics, 21(5):949–965.

Vehvilainen, L.M., Zielstorff, R., Gertman, P.M., Tzeng, M.C., Estey, G. (2002). Alzheimer's Caregiver Internet Support System (ACISS): Evaluating the Feasibility and Effectiveness of Supporting Family Caregivers Virtually. American Medical Informatics Association 2002 Symposium, 11 November 2002. S32 Poster Session 1.

White, M.H., Dorman, S.M. (2000) Online support for caregivers: Analysis of an internet Alzheimer mailgroup. Computers in Nursing, 18:168–176.

Wilson, B.A., Emslie, H.C., Quirk, K., Evans, J.J. (2001) Reducing everyday memory and planning problems by means of a paging system: A randomised control crossover study. Journal of Neurology, Neurosurgery and Psychiatry, 70:477–482.

Winslow, B.W. (2003) Family caregivers' experiences with community services: A qualitative analysis. Public Health in Nursing, 20:341–348.

Woolham, J. (2005). Safe at Home. The effectiveness of assistive technology in supporting the independence of people with dementia: The Safe at Home project. Hawker Publications, London.

Yasuda, K., Beckman, B., Yoneda, M., Yoneda, H., Iwamoto, A., Nakamura, T. (2006) Successful guidance by automatic output of music and verbal messages for daily behavioural disturbances of three individuals with dementia. Neuropsychological Rehabilation, 16:66–82.

Zanetti, O., Zanieri, G., Vreese, L.Pd., Frisoni, G.B., Binetti, G., Trabucchi, M. (2000). Utilizing an electronic memory aid with Alzheimer's disease patients. A study of feasibility. Paper presented at the 6th International Stockholm/Springfield Symposium on Advances in Alzheimer Therapy.

Chapter 5
Assistive Technologies and Issues Relating to Privacy, Ethics and Security

Suzanne Martin, Johan E. Bengtsson, and Rose-Marie Dröes

Abstract Emerging technologies provide the opportunity to develop innovative sustainable service models, capable of supporting adults with dementia at home. Devices range from simple stand-alone components that can generate a responsive alarm call to complex interoperable systems that even can be remotely controlled. From these complex systems the paradigm of the ubiquitous or ambient smart home has emerged, integrating technology, environmental design and traditional care provision. The service context is often complex, involving a variety of stakeholders and a range of interested agencies. Against this backdrop, as anecdotal evidence and government policies spawn further innovation it is critical that due consideration is given to the potential ethical ramifications at an individual, organisational and societal level. Well-grounded ethical thinking and proactive ethical responses to this innovation are required. Explicit policy and practice should therefore emerge which engenders confidence in existing supported living option schemes for adults with dementia and informs further innovation.

5.1 Introduction

For the person with dementia, information and communication technologies (ICT) can support community-based alternatives to long-term institutional care (Hughes 2002; Baldwin 2005). As disease progression adversely affects individual cognition, functional ability may decrease and risk scenarios for the individual increase. Technological devices potentially have a strong and positive role to play as part of an integrated supported living option. Within this paradigm ethical issues emerge

S. Martin (✉)
TRAIL Living Lab, School of Health Sciences, Faculty of Life and Health Sciences, University of Ulster, Jordanstown, Northern Ireland
e-mail: s.martin@ulster.ac.uk

M.D. Mulvenna, C.D. Nugent (eds.), *Supporting People with Dementia Using Pervasive Health Technologies*, Advanced Information and Knowledge Processing, DOI 10.1007/978-1-84882-551-2_5, © Springer-Verlag London Limited 2010

which require sound thinking to generate robust policies and secure systems to underpin practice and ensure privacy.

Whilst technology items per se can be considered as "neutral" devices, the application within services generates care scenarios that are often complex. Within these complex scenarios ethical issues can occur when technology is used as an intervention in the life of the person with dementia. Major concerns are the right for protection of personal data (privacy), the rights of the elderly, and integration of persons with disabilities (Stanford Encyclopaedia of Philosophy 2005). For any intervention, the principles of free and informed consent of the person concerned must be respected, taking also into account that persons with dementia should be assumed to be vulnerable (Stanford Encyclopaedia of Philosophy 2005).

Information security must be built into any assistive technology to ensure confidentiality (privacy), data integrity, availability and accountability. In particular personal information must be stored securely, and devices for accessing this information must be secured against unauthorised access to information.

Finally, ethics, privacy and security are not possible unless the system fulfils some basic quality criteria. Of particular concern is providing functionality corresponding to user needs, usability to ensure that the needs can be fulfilled, and reliability to ensure that the system is available, does not have security weaknesses and adheres to agreed quality assurance protocols such as ISO 9126-1 quality assurance for software engineering.

5.2 Technology Options from a User Perspective

This chapter presents information on a wide spectrum of technologies that are, or will be, commercially available to support adults with dementia. These range from single stand-alone devices to fully networked integrated systems. Various contributors have suggested ways to conceptualise the technology components, most of which assume a technology perspective. For example, Dard (1996) focuses on the flow of information within the home, Barlow and Gann (1998) concentrate on the technology and Jedamizik (2001) emphasises the control and information available to the user. Aldrich (2003) proposes a hierarchical classification, from the users perspective, which retains a focus on the functionality of the technology. Various levels of communication attainable are highlighted and differentiation between systems is affirmed between those systems which can learn from those that can't; and those systems which retain a constant awareness of tenants and those that don't. The Table 5.1 below outlines the five hierarchical classifications and the devices and applications emerging within social care.

Within literature diverse terms are applied when disseminating information relating to technology use for people with dementia. On occasions a technology descriptor is used as in *social alarms* or *preventative technology*, whilst sometimes a descriptor for the resulting service applications is applied, for example, *smart homes, telecare, context aware home*, and the *ubiquitous home*. It is possible that

Table 5.1 Five hierarchical classes of smart home (Aldrich 2003)

Classification	Description	Application
1. Homes which contain intelligent objects	Single stand-alone appliances and objects which function in an intelligent manner	Talking calendars; big button picture telephones http://www.atdementia.org.uk
2. Homes containing intelligent communicating objects	Appliances and objects function intelligently and may exchange information between one another to increase functionality	Hillmount Close Supported living option for people with acquired head injury and complex physical disability http://www.cedar-foundation.org
3. Connected homes	Internal and external networks may be present allowing interactive and remote control of systems. Access to services and information from both within and beyond the home may be facilitated	Sydenham Court technology enriched supported living option for people with dementia, Belfast Northern Ireland
4. Learning homes	Patterns of activity in the home are recorded and the accumulated data are used to anticipate user needs and to control the technology	Adaptive Home Colorado http://www.cs.colorado.edu/~mozer/house
5. Attentive homes	Activity and location of people and objects within the homes are constantly registered and this information is used to control technology in anticipation of the occupants needs	The Aware Home Colorado http://www.awarehome.gatech.edu/

two similar services integrating the same technological components are described in very different ways! This can be confusing when trying to source information to assist with service innovation and development.

5.3 Ethics

Ethics can be described as the constructed norms of internal consistency regarding what is right and what is wrong. From this a systematic reasoning of how we ought to act in a given situation should emerge, where reasoning is guided by our internal values and morals, the expectation of wider society and the codes of ethics that govern professional practice. Dubois and Miley (1996) suggest a distinction between microethics (principles and standards that direct individual practice) and macroethics (which deal with organisational arrangements and social policy).

Ethical theories encourage consideration of dilemmas from differing perspectives. Dentological theories of ethics suggest that interventions should be considered in relation to pre-existing duty-based requirements within the given scenario. Within this paradigm the measure of rightness or wrongness of an action is not considered in relation to the consequences it evokes. Legislation often supports the dentological approach, consider, for example, the values embedded within the articles of the European convention on Human Rights; right to life is protected by law, no one shall be subjected to inhuman or degrading treatment, everyone has the right to liberty and security, everyone has the right to respect for private family life, home and correspondence.

In contrast consequentialist theories suggest that in reflecting on the ethical aspects of a scenario the consequences of the action should assist with decision making. Within this approach *ethical egoism* suggests that an action is morally right if the overall consequences are favourable for the person carrying out the action; *ethical altruism* considers the consequences for everyone except the person carrying out the action.

Hughes and Baldwin (2006) suggest that when considering ethical issues in relation to dementia care, rather than choose between a theoretical approach, it is appropriate to take a principle-based approach. The principals that should inform ethical practice in this subject area stem from the four principles of medical ethics (after Bjørneby et al. 1999):

- Autonomy: people should be able to decide what they want to happen or be done to them.
- Beneficence: we should try to do good to the people we care for.
- Non-maleficence: we should try to avoid doing people harm.
- Justice: people should be treated fairly and equally.

5.4 Privacy

Privacy as a concept is neither clearly understood nor easily defined and yet the fear of a loss of personal privacy, specifically related to information and communication technology receives a lot of media attention (Tavani 2007). Specific concerns relate to the amount of personal information that is gathered, the speed it is transported (raising concerns about its accuracy), the duration of time that personal information is stored and also the kind of information to be transferred. Tavani (2007) summaries three views of privacy as

1. Accessibility privacy: which is physically being left alone or being free from intrusion into your physical space.
2. Decisional privacy: relates to the freedom to make personal choices and decisions.
3. Informational privacy: which concerns control over the flow of personal information, including the transfer and exchange of information.

Moore (2000) considers that an individual has privacy in a particular situation if they are protected from intrusion, interference and information access by others. It becomes possible to differentiate between having the right to privacy and having privacy in when particular conditions are satisfied. Moore also states that privacy is an outward expression of the core value and personal desire for security.

To protect the privacy of the user of assistive technology, the aim of assistive technology and the way it is used by service providers or care organisations, as well as how personal data will be handled by care personnel and processed electronically, must be described explicitly in a privacy statement and communicated to the user.

The privacy statement should include the name and function of the person who has final responsibility for the daily processing of the personal data; the location where the data are stored in paper and/or electronic form; the specific aim, content and usage of the data and the person(s) who informs the user about this; the person(s) that can be contacted if personal data prove to be incorrect; and measures that are taken to prevent inspection, mutation or removal of data by unauthorised persons.

Personal data should be processed only after explicit informed consent of the user. Access to personal information, and sharing with other professionals involved in the care provision, should be well controlled, with protective measures explicitly articulated to the person with dementia and – to a varying degree – the informal carer(s) (Martin et al. 2007). Consent to such access and sharing of information can be given, withheld or withdrawn at any time. Situations of non-consensual disclosure of personal information must be highlighted to the person with dementia and their carers and the point of seeking consent to use the device or service. It must be clearly stated in which scenarios or situations this would be deemed to be a necessity, and how this decision is reached weighed against attendant risks of non-disclosure.

Additional measures to recommend are to store personal data in devices only if necessary for the goal of assistance or care and for as long as necessary, then deleting them or transferring them to a secure central location if there is reasonable expectation that the user will benefit from it in the (near) future.

5.5 Security

Computer security has been defined as having three elements of confidentiality (protecting against unauthorised disclosure of information to third parties), integrity (preventing unauthorised modification of data and files) and availability (preventing unauthorised withholding of information from those who need it when they need it) (Kizza 2003). The concepts of privacy and security are often linked. Security issues can be considered under three broad categories:

1. Data security – which is either resident in or exchanged between computer systems
2. System security – relating to hardware and software

3. Network security – including networks and the internet (Spinello and Tavani 2004; Tavani 2007).

Making technological systems secure is a complex task and should therefore be done in a systematic manner; for example, following standards such as ISO-17799, used as a code of practice for information security management. When developing and field testing pervasive healthcare services and technologies for people with dementia, the main security themes to consider are System Access Control, Computer & Network Management, Security Organisation, and a Security Policy that ensures Compliance with regulations and user requirements. In addition, good practice for systems development and risk analysis should be used.

Healthcare systems for people with dementia will be accessed by different stakeholders, for example, carers (staff and relatives), the persons with dementia themselves and technicians. Access should be protected by strong passwords or better mechanisms. The person with dementia presents a special difficulty, as requiring a password would be difficult for them to remember and use. Therefore automated authentication methods must be considered, for example wearing a wireless authentication badge or face recognition.

All computer and network equipment must be protected from theft and misuse. In particular computers in the home must not retain the sensitive personal data of the person with dementia any longer than absolutely necessary, deleting it, making it inaccessible or transferring it to a central secure storage. All communication between physical nodes must be strongly encrypted.

A security policy should be created that ensures that ethics and privacy issues are respected, and that information security is not breached. A security sub-group could be created that checks that the security policy is not violated, and assists personnel involved in the operation of services to maintain security.

Schneier (2004) considers it appropriate to view security as a process not a product of the technology. He argues that risk assessment is key to this process and that attaining perfect security would in effect render a system useless. This is contrary to the view of Kizza (2003) who considers that complete security can be achieved if mechanisms for deterrence, prevention, detection and response are in place.

5.6 Discussion on Ethical Practice and Technology Use

Ethical issues clearly exist in the use of technology with people who have dementia. As stated previously technology devices are neutral; however, the integration into care scenarios for people with dementia makes it complex. Whilst this could be argued for all services that utilise technology the confounding factor when supporting adults with dementia is the altered cognitive capacity of the person receiving the service. Within the legal framework supporting service developments/delivery and the generic rights of citizens within democratic societies it is therefore crucial that ethical concerns are debated thoroughly and resolved in a transparent manner.

At an organisational level it is crucial that the use of technology to support people with dementia is informed by an ethical framework, which is translated into explicit organisational policies and procedures, informed by legislation and national policy. This activity needs to be undertaken in advance of thinking about what products or systems could be used. Organisations need to educate and empower their staff for the responsibilities of using technology and think through how it is to function in the care model.

All practicable efforts to seek informed consent should be sought. The different stages of the dementia condition, variance in cognitive function, the environment (Day et al. 2000) and even the time of day (Jacques and Jackson 2000) can affect the individual's capacity to understand and consent to a particular intervention. However, it is unacceptable not to have ensured that all efforts have been taken to seek consent and provide information to the person with dementia, unless this right has been designated to another person (Bartlett 2005).

Evidence exists to demonstrate that people with dementia are repeatedly excluded from consultation about aspects of their care (Allan 2001; Clare 2004). A predominant culture remains within which what people with dementia say is viewed as unreliable or lacking content (Weiner et al. 1999). The move towards consulting and listening to people with dementia is slow and involves changing from an emphasis on the pathology of the condition to the potential of the individual (Reid et al. 2001; Dröes 2007). If consent is to be really sought from the person with dementia then the organisation seeking to use an assistive technology must have ensured that staff are trained in a range of communication methods; otherwise the person with dementia has been denied their rights.

The ethical framework applied to the use of assistive technology in dementia care cannot be limited to the care organisation or individual responsible for a piece of equipment. The technology companies who make and supply devices also carry ethical responsibility for their practice. Technology products can at times appear to be a quick and easy solution to a problem. A technology company has an ethical responsibility to fully inform those considering a purchase of the possible implications of use. In the context of people with dementia, an ethical technology company should seek to find out what the problem is and support the customer in thinking about all the possible solutions before encouraging the sale of an assistive technology.

5.6.1 Explicitness, Legal and Procedural Context

The prevalence of supported living environments with embedded technology to support older people with cognitive impairment is increasing. At the meso/macro level the coordinating organisation should be explicit how electronic assistive technology is used within care options. The aims and objectives of using such technology need to be explicit and the legal and procedural context in which it can be considered also needs to be understood.

5.6.2 Person-Centred Approach

It is preferable that a person centred approach to care is followed and it should be an easy assessment process to identify all the tenant's care needs and why assistive technology is being considered. These points are very important, especially with equipment that is monitoring or gathering data on a person. The use of technology should not be considered as a separate part of an individual's care, but additional to the care offered by professionals and integrated into the overall care planning process.

5.6.3 Care Staff Training

At an operational level care staff need to be trained in how to care for and respond to people with dementia and how the technology is integrated into the care process. Approaches to supporting the person with dementia need to be well established. For example, in some home-based caring scenarios rather than have a sensor switch to disable the cooker at all times, support staff could either check after meal times that the cooker has been switched off or provide a member of staff to accompany the vulnerable older person during meal preparation if required.

Location technology has been used both in the community and institutional care settings for people with dementia. "Tagging" is at times still used as a term to describe this or similar devices. This technology can be used in a variety of ways; it can alert the care provider if the vulnerable person is approaching an exit to leave the building, it could enable staff to locate the person if he or she is out, unattended, in an agreed area. This may well enable the older person to remain an independent walker; however, it could also be that on occasions the person is amenable to be accompanied when walking. Tagging technology is one that has attracted substantial adverse media publicity (Clarke and Keady 2002). The risks associated with independent walking to the user may be high. Based on the recent evidence, it has been established that nearly 25% of people in care homes who "wander" experience a fatal or serious injury (Stanford Encyclopaedia of Philosophy 2005). On the other side fall incidents can also be diminished when, e.g. during the night, assistive technology alerts the caregiver to offer support to the elderly person who goes to the bathroom (Lauriks et al. 2008). A blended approach to technology integration into care seems to be a more appropriate approach, rather than a prescriptive application in all scenarios.

5.6.4 Protection and Paternalism

The theories of ethics, and principles of good practice outlined above can help to establish a good ethical approach to services, as they provide both an organisational macro-ethical framework and consider issues in relation to the individual. However, how can these issues be adequately considered if the service user either doesn't or hasn't the mental capacity to consent to technology use as part of her care package?

Is it then justified for the care providers or relatives to promote this approach on the basis that the individual will be better off living in this supported housing scheme (rather than institutional care), or that the technology will ensure the person will be better protected from harm?

This raises the issue of "paternalism" which is the interference of a state or individual in relation to another person, either against their will or when the interference is justified by a claim of better protection for the individual. This is important in applying ethics into situations of reduced cognitive capacity. Does a trade-off exist with regard to the desire to put in place best practice to benefit the welfare of the service user and their right to make their own decisions?

Dworkin suggests that certain conditions can be considered when aiming to establish if paternalism is present (Stanford Encyclopaedia of Philosophy 2005). These conditions concern the service user (X), the care provider (Y) and the use of technology (Z).

- Does the application (or omission) of technology (Z) interfere with the liberty or autonomy of the service user (X)?
- Does the care provider (Y) use technology without the consent of the service user (X)?
- Does the care provider (Y) use the technology (Z) because of a belief that it will improve the welfare of the service user (X)?

Can the care provider demonstrate that the use of tagging technology doesn't limit the liberty or autonomy of the user rather than justifying its use under both a duty-based approach to care and considering the consequences of not using available technology? Is paternalism always wrong? Is it plausible that paternalism in the case of some individual users is acceptable when the act of using the technology is intended for their benefit? In this instance it is crucial that the means by which ethical issues are addressed and the good brought to the service user can be highlighted.

Paternalism aims to protect people from themselves, assuming their safety is more important than their liberty. This contrasts with "harm principle" suggested by Mill which cites that limiting liberty can only be justified to prevent harm to others, not self harm although this can only be applied in circumstances of clear cognitive ability.

It is conceivable that a paternalistic approach emerges as the predominant ethos within a technology enriched supported living option for people with dementia, if attempts are not made to establish the individuals' beliefs and values in relation to living in this type of care model. How then can the care provider clearly demonstrate application of the four principles of medical ethics described above?

5.6.5 Information, Demonstration and Individual Consent

Consider then again a service user who is planning to move from home to a supported living option. It would be good practice for this person and his or her main family/carers to visit the facility beforehand. A prearranged visit provides the opportunity to experience the living space, meet with staff, other residents and see the technology on offer. At this point service staff could give the user information on the facility, outline technology on offer and specify why it is used. An individualised profile of preferred assistive technology might also be discussed. The provided information should capture both the organisational ethical approach, and in layman's terms explain the ethical approach used in relation to individual service users.

Information could be provided in printed copy to take home, and a demonstration of the technology in use should be available during their visit. Scenarios of technology use could also help clarify the potential of the devices and the consequences of their use; for example, the benefit of a picture phone which may enable independent contact with close family members. However, for the relative it could also generate a high volume of calls on a regular, unmonitored level if memory problems result in the user forgetting previous contact.

In relation to the sensor data that are gathered the operational implementation of this could be explained. How the data are kept safe, so that privacy is guaranteed, who has access to the computer system, and who has the authority to alter sensor functions or generate reports. It should be clearly explained how the data will be used, and when it will be shared with other professionals involved in care provision. Again scenarios can be used to explain this to both the user and her family so they fully understand how the technology is integrated into the overall care process. A discussion on the importance of consenting to live in the type of supported living option could be initiated at this point, to include highlighting implications for the service user and her family as cognitive capacity declines. In relation to this it should also be explicitly discussed with the persons with dementia and their carers that assistive technology cannot prevent people with dementia from all problems and risks that are a consequence of the disease (such as dangerous behaviour, falls, wandering at night, disorientation). This means that risk factors associated with the disease and with the execution of daily activities will be prevalent, also with the use of assistive technology.

Kurzweill (2005) suggested the ELSI (Ethical, Legal, Social Implications) model as guidance to the development of an ethical framework to guide researchers. However, others (Weckbert and Moore 2004) consider that this ethics-first approach may have problems as it requires thorough determination of the specific harms a technology may do in advance, arguing (specifically in relation to nanotechnologies) that a continually reflection on ethical implication is required.

5.7 Summary and Conclusions

Ethical issues abound in all aspects of interventions to support adults with dementia. Whilst technology may have a positive role to play in supporting people with dementia, it may not be appropriate for all individuals, or it might only be considered for some individuals, some of the time.

Organisations should give ethical consideration to using technology enriched care provision to reflect both organisational ethos and the service approach at an individual level. If an organisation is to use assistive technology they need to have informed policies and procedures using an ethical framework that is defined by their national legislation on the protection of the rights of citizens with dementia. Such a policy must be integrated to the overall care approach and not be considered as a separate intervention. If such structures are in place then technologies are more likely to be used to positively support the lives of people with dementia avoiding a paternalistic delivery of care.

Acknowledgements The authors acknowledge the contribution of Professor Chris Nugent, and Mr Colm Cunningham to an original article, which informed this chapter (Martin et al. 2007).

Appendix: Checklists to Assist Using Technology with People Who Have Dementia

When technology is used checks need to be in place that ensures the following questions are addressed:

- Has consent been sought from the person with dementia about the use of technology in their care, using skilled personnel and appropriate communication methods?
- Has a date been set to review the use of this technology intervention? Is it accepted by the user and does it support the care process?
- On what aspects is the effectiveness of the assistive technology in the care of the person evaluated and by what methods?

For Professionals and Field Test Personnel

- Professional carers and system administrators must have knowledge of key principles of healthcare confidentiality: privacy, explicit or implicit consent, and conditions for non-consensual disclosure.
- Since persons with dementia are vulnerable, they shall be given all necessary support to understand the confidentiality issues and express their wishes. The individual's ability to understand, retain and weigh up information as well as communicate their decision should be examined.
- The consent should be given until end-of-service, i.e. until end of user test, death or explicit withdrawal of consent, so that the consent also covers later stages in the disease when the person with dementia might be incapable of giving consent.
- Personally identifiable data shall be deleted and made non-recoverable on the test equipment as part of uninstallation.
- Using staff from other agencies requires explicit consent and possibly formal information protection agreements.
- Necessary secondary uses of information (for example, for payments or management) requires explicit consent.

- The basis for the configuration of the device should at all times be the subjective needs and wants of the person with mild dementia.
- The benefits of information sharing with the informal carer should be discussed with the person with dementia.
- In emergency situations minimum necessary confidential user information may be used or disclosed.
- Confidential data relating to persons with dementia shall be stored on secure computers, with up-to-date protections against unauthorised access and malware.

For Developers

- Security analyses should be performed at unit and system levels. It should be performed at the specification stage, and as part of evaluation. The security analysis should address requirements for confidentiality, data integrity, availability and accountability. It should specifically analyse malware threats and the potential for system abuse by users.
- An authorisation model should be defined so that any access to identifiable personal data is strictly controlled. Person with dementia access should be made by means of implicit or automatic device authentication. Accesses by all other users (e.g. carers, researchers and administrators) should require user-level authentication.
- A service model should be defined so that the persons with dementia and their carers can be informed of what kinds of information is being recorded and for what purposes.
- Build the system so that it minimises the potential to stigmatise the user. This means that devices should preferably be perceived and used as normal technology artefacts, also by people that do not suffer from dementia.
- There must be a generic way to access stored data, for system administrators (for research, emergency or legal purposes), and for the person with dementia's access to own stored data (as guaranteed by Data Protection laws).
- Data should be stored with as little identifying information as possible. If possible, the system should be partitioned into one part where identifiable personal data exist, and other parts where it is impossible to trace to which physical person some data belong.
- The personal codes that are used in data collection for research purposes, must NOT be reused in the normal operation of the system.
- Only near-future data should be cached in other nodes than where the original data reside.
- Data that are not needed anymore for the operation of the system should immediately be made inaccessible.[1]

---

[1]By deleting the data, or by one-way encryption where decryption keys are stored in external protected systems.

- All communication links should be secure. Encrypted files and databases must be used for storing identifiable personal data.

For Researchers

- Researchers that execute the evaluation of the prototype with user dyads shall have no business dependencies themselves with commercial organisations within or outside the project consortium.
- Personally identifiable data must be stored in encoded form.
- Mapping collected data to individuals must use keys stored separately in locked closets.
- Only encoded data will be transmitted between sites.
- Be sensitive to the changing clinical phases of dementia that may influence the subjects' autonomy and capacity.
- Under no circumstances permit reporting of details during dissemination that would allow the identification of any subject involved.

References

Aldrich, F. (2003) Smart homes: Past, present and future. In: Harper R., (eds.) Inside the Smart Home. Springer Verlag, London, England.

Allan, K. (2001) Communication and Consultation. Exploring Ways for Staff to Involve People with Dementia in Developing Services. The Policy Press, Bristol, UK.

Baldwin, C. (2005) Technology, dementia and ethics: Rethinking the issues. Disability Studies Quarterly, 25:3.

Barlow, J., Gann, D. 1998. A changing sense of place: Are integrated IT systems reshaping the home? Technologies Future, Urban Features Conference, Durham, 23–24 April.

Bartlett, P. (2005) Blackstone's Guide to the Mental Capacity Act. Oxford University Press, UK.

Bjornrby, S., Topo, P., Holthe, T. (1999) Technology, Ethics and Dementia: A Guidebook on How to Apply Technology in Dementia Care. The Norwegian Centre for Dementia Research, INFO-Bank, Norway.

Clarke, C., Keady, J. (2002) Getting down to brass tacks: A discussion of data collection with people with dementia. In: H. Wilkinson (eds.) The Perspectives of People with Dementia: Research Methods and Motivations. Jessica Kingsley Publishers, London, England.

Clare, L. (2004) Awareness in early-stage Alzheimer's disease: A review of methods and evidence. British Journal of Clinical Psychology, 43(Pt 2):177–196.

Dard, P. 1996. Dilemmas of Telesurveillance in Housing. ENHR Housing Conference, Helsingor.

Day, K., Carreon, D., Stump, C. (2000) The therapeutic design of environments for people with dementia: A review of the empirical research. The Gerontological Society of America, 40: 397–416.

Dröes, R.M. (2007) Insight in coping with dementia; listening to the voice of those who suffer from it. Aging and Mental Health, 11(2):115–118.

Dubois, B., Miley, K. (1996) Social Work: An Empowering Profession. Allyn and Bacon, Harlow.

Dworkin, G. (2005) Paternalism. In: Stanford Encyclopedia of Philosophy. Available at http://plato.stanford.edu/entries/paternalism/, Accessed on April 18 2007.

Hughes, J. (2002) Electronic tagging of people with dementia who wander: Ethical issues are possibly more important than practical benefits. British Medical Journal, 325:847–848.

Hughes, J., Baldwin, C. (2006) Ethical Issues in Dementia Care. Jessica Kingsley Publishers, London, England.

Jacques, A., Jackson, G. (2000) Understanding Dementia, 3rd edn. Churchill Livingstone, Edinburgh.

Jedamizik, M. (2001) Smart House: A Usable Dialog System for the Control of Technical Systems by Gesture Recognition in Home Environments. Available at http://is7-www.cs.umi-dortmund.de/research/gesture/argus/intelligent-home.html, accessed on 23.12.08.

Kizza, J. (2003) Ethical and Social Issues in the Information Age, 2nd edn. Springer-Verlag, New York.

Kurzweill, R. (2005) Nanoscience, nanotechnology and ethics: Promise or peril. In: H. Tavani (ed.) Ethics and Technology: Ethical Issues in an Age of Information and Communication Technology, 2nd edn. John Wiley and Sons, USA, p. 375.

Lauriks, S., Osté, J., Hertogh, C.M.P.M., Dröes, R.M. (2008) Meer levenskwaliteit met domotica (More Quality of Life in Smart Homes). VU University Medical Center, Department of Psychiatry, Amsterdam.

Martin, S., Cunningham, C., Nugent, C. (2007) Ethical considerations for integrating technology into community based service models for adults with dementia. Alzheimer's Care Today, 8(3):251–259.

Moore, J. (2000) Towards a theory of privacy for the information age. In: H. Tavani (ed.) Ethics and Technology: Ethical Issues in an Age of Information and Communication Technology, 2nd edn. John Wiley and Sons, USA.

Reid, D., Ryan, T., Enderby, P. (2001) What does it mean to listen to people with dementia?. Disability and Society, 16(3):377–392.

Schneier, B. (2004) Secrets and lies: Digital security in a networked world. In: Tavani, H. (ed.) Ethics and Technology: Ethical Issues in an Age of Information and Communication Technology, 2nd edn. John Wiley and Sons, USA, p. 189.

Spinello, R.A., Tavani, H.T. (2004) In: H. Tavani (ed.) Ethics and Technology: Ethical Issues in an Age of Information and Communication Technology, 2nd edn. John Wiley and Sons, USA, p. 171.

Tavani, H. (2007) Ethics and Technology: Ethical Issues in an Age of Information and Communication Technology, 2nd edn. John Wiley and Sons, USA.

Weiner, D., Peterson, B., Keefe, F. (1999) Chronic pain-associated behaviours in the nursing home: Resident versus caregiver perceptions. Pain – International Association for the Study of Pain, 80:577–588.

Weckbert, J., Moore, J. (2004) Using the precautionary principle in nanotechnology. In: H. Tavani (ed.) Ethics and Technology: Ethical Issues in an Age of Information and Communication Technology, 2nd edn. John Wiley and Sons, USA, p. 376.

Part II
The Role of the User in the Design Process

Chapter 6
Identifying User Needs and the Participative Design Process

Franka Meiland, Rose-Marie Dröes, Stefan Sävenstedt, Birgitta Bergvall-Kåreborn, and Anna-Lena Andersson

Abstract As the number of persons with dementia increases and also the demands on care and support at home, additional solutions to support persons with dementia are needed. The COGKNOW project aims to develop an integrated, user-driven cognitive prosthetic device to help persons with dementia. The project focuses on support in the areas of memory, social contact, daily living activities and feelings of safety. The design process is user-participatory and consists of iterative cycles at three test sites across Europe. In the first cycle persons with dementia and their carers ($n = 17$) actively participated in the developmental process. Based on their priorities of needs and solutions, on their disabilities and after discussion between the team, a top four list of Information and Communication Technology (ICT) solutions was made and now serves as the basis for development: in the area of remembering – day and time orientation support, find mobile service and reminding service, in the area of social contact – telephone support by picture dialling, in the area of daily activities – media control support through a music playback and radio function, and finally, in the area of safety – a warning service to indicate when the front door is open and an emergency contact service to enhance feelings of safety. The results of this first project phase show that, in general, the people with mild dementia as well as their carers were able to express and prioritize their (unmet) needs, and the kind of technological assistance they preferred in the selected areas. In next phases it will be tested if the user-participatory design and multidisciplinary approach employed in the COGKNOW project result in a user-friendly, useful device that positively impacts the autonomy and quality of life of persons with dementia and their carers.

F. Meiland (✉)
Department of Psychiatry, Alzheimer Centre, VU University Medical Centre/GGZ Buitenamstel, Amsterdam, The Netherlands
e-mail: fj.meiland@vumc.nl

Large parts of this chapter are reprinted with permission of Nova Science Publishers, Inc. from Non-pharmacological Therapies in Dementia, vol. 1, 2010, User-participatory development of assistive technology for people with dementia – from needs to functional requirements. First results of the COGKNOW project, F.J.M. Meiland, A. Reinersmann, S. Sävenstedt, et al.

6.1 Introduction

One of the great challenges of the twenty-first century will be the provision of adequate care to the growing number of elderly people, and in particular, those with dementia. With an estimated number of 24 million people world-wide suffering from dementia at present (Ferri et al. 2005), a number expected to double every 20 years, health care systems require significant adaptation to meet the future demands of persons with dementia.

Already, nursing homes and long-term care facilities face enormous shortcomings in the recruitment of adequately trained staff. Health care economies are increasingly aware of the financial demands required to provide quality care for people suffering from dementia. Official policies therefore aim to enable people with dementia to stay at home as long as possible, which is what they themselves want (Health Council, Netherlands 2002). However, community dwelling people with dementia very often receive insufficient care and are largely dependent on informal carers for the provision of care that is not covered by formal services (Health Council, Netherlands 2002).

Research focusing on the needs of people with dementia indicates that formal services primarily meet needs involved in supporting basic activities of daily living (ADL): washing, dressing and feeding the person with dementia whereas other individual needs are largely neglected. Community dwelling people with dementia hence suffer from various unmet needs for which currently support is not provided. Subjective reports of people with dementia living in the community predominantly indicate unmet needs in the areas of memory, company, psychological distress, daily activities and information (van der Roest et al. 2007). Support of needs in these areas is of high importance to them and can contribute to their well-being and quality of life. Well-being and quality of life in turn positively influence health and behavioural symptoms as well as admission to nursing homes and mortality rates (Gaugler et al. 2005). The higher the degree of unmet needs by formal services, the higher the burden for the informal carer and the more likely is an admission to a nursing home early in the illness process (Gaugler et al. 2005).

Without changes in current health care systems, even the current standards, in which at least part of the needs are met, cannot be maintained. In addition, given the rapid growth of people suffering from dementia and the parallel decrease in the number of persons of the working population who are potentially available to offer formal and informal care, the unmet needs of people with dementia will grow even to a greater extent.

Finding alternative strategies to provide high quality yet cost-effective care services that enable people with dementia to remain at home, in a safe and acceptable manner, is therefore of vital importance.

One possible solution is the greater use of assistive technology, an umbrella term for different technological systems and devices that can assist people who have functional limitations due to age-related disabilities such as dementia (ASTRID 2000). Assistive technology can offer a cost-effective means to enhance independency and quality of life in people with dementia as well as enable them to remain in their own environment, which is what they themselves generally prefer (Health Council, Netherlands 2002). The potential role of these new technologies in health care is recognized (ASTRID 2000) but so far, there has been limited exploitation of the opportunities they present to support older people with dementia in their everyday lives (ASTRID 2000). A reason for the limited application of assistive technology for people with dementia is the complexity of the device in a forgetful and dyspraxic and often heterogeneous group (Orpwood et al. 2005). General research into product development of assistive technology demonstrates usability and user-friendliness as the main factors for cost-effective production and acceptance by the end-user (Andersson et al. 2002; Cohene et al. 2005). In many instances, currently available applications or devices for people with dementia have been designed by professional organizations with little involvement of the end-user, the person with dementia (Orpwood et al. 2005).

Dementia affects every individual differently and each person has his own specific set of circumstances, disabilities and needs. The individual's requirements when it comes to providing a supporting technology are similarly wide-ranging. Development processes are therefore probably best pursued where technological experts and those experienced in the needs of persons with dementia act in tandem with a user-participatory developmental design process, engaging groups of persons with dementia and their carers from the start. That way, difficulties related to lack of insight and technological naivety in this group of mostly older persons are approached in a combined fashion, and the heterogeneous functional requirements of this special group are ascertained in the most suitable way. Knowledge about abilities and disabilities of the person with dementia and context information on living arrangements provide essential information in this regard (ASTRID 2000; Hagen et al. 2002; Nygard and Starkhammar 2007). However, of even greater importance is clear information on user-needs and preferences, as these determine whether the person with dementia will perceive the device as useful and thus influence the extent of future engagement (ASTRID 2000; Nygard and Starkhammar 2007; Nugent 2007). A thorough needs assessment to learn more about the actual needs and wishes of people with dementia regarding Information and Communication Technology (ICT) solutions is therefore indispensable.

The need to involve the person with dementia in the development process motivated the COGKNOW project. COGKNOW is a 3 year, European Framework Programme project in which integrated, user-participatory, ICT solutions are developed to help people with mild dementia navigate through their day. The project focuses on need areas in which earlier research from one of the consortium partners (VU University medical centre) identified most unmet needs, namely memory support, social contact, daily activities and feelings of safety (Dröes et al. 2005; van der Roest et al. 2007, 2009).

In this chapter, we report on the needs and ICT solutions inventory that was carried out among people with dementia and their carers in the first phase of the COGKNOW project (Hettinga et al. 2007). The needs and preferred ICT solutions inventory focused on the following research questions:

- What concrete needs do people with mild dementia and their carers express in the areas of memory, communication, daily activities and psychological distress?
- Do people with mild dementia and their carer prefer specific ICT solutions to address their needs?
- Taking into account the needs, abilities, context variables and preferences of people with mild dementia and their carers, which ICT device(s) could possibly provide adequate solutions for their wishes?

6.2 Method

6.2.1 Design

The user-participatory design process consists of three iterative cycles in a 3-year time period (2006–2009). In each cycle 12–18 community dwelling persons with mild dementia and their carers, spread out over three test sites (Amsterdam, Belfast and Luleå), are invited to participate in the study. Thus, in total about 45 persons with mild dementia and their carers will participate in the study. Each cycle starts with an inventory among the participants of user needs and preferred ICT solutions in the selected support areas of the COGKNOW project by means of workshops and (standardized) interviews. In principle, separate workshops are organized for people with dementia and carers, to give them the opportunity to express their own opinion. In addition to the workshops, domiciliary individual interviews are conducted using standardized questionnaires to collect information that could be relevant in developing an ICT solution, such as personal background and context characteristics, cognitive functioning (disabilities), (unmet) needs and experienced autonomy. The results of the workshops and interviews are used as input for the (further) technological development of the device. Each cycle ends with user field tests in which the developed prototype is tested with people with dementia, and a thorough, so-called human factors impact analysis is carried out on the user-friendliness, usefulness and (in the last iteration also on) the impact of the prototype on the daily life of people with dementia and their carers. In this way participants contribute to the design process as well as to the implementation and evaluation process.

The study was approved by the relevant medical ethical authority of each research site.

6.2.2 Sample and Setting

In the first project phase 17 people with mild dementia of the Alzheimer type and their carers were recruited from memory clinics and/or the Meeting Centres Support Programme for people with dementia and their carers in Amsterdam (VUmc), Belfast (BCH) and Luleå (CDH/NLL). At every research site, five to six patient–carer dyads were recruited.

Inclusion criteria that were

- People with a diagnosis of dementia of the Alzheimer type (possible/probable) as described in the DSM-IV-TR
- Severity of dementia: global deterioration stage 3, 4, 5: mild cognitive decline (early confusional; GDS 3) moderate cognitive decline (late confusional; GDS 4) and moderately severe cognitive decline (early dementia; GDS 5) (assessed by using the standardized Brief Cognitive Rating Scale (Reisberg et al. 1982))
- People are willing and able to participate actively (through individual interviews, participation in a small focus group and field test sessions) in a research project in which an ICT device is being developed that aims to support them in their memory, daily activities, social contact with family and friends and feelings of safety
- The informal carer has regular contact with/cares for the person with dementia.

6.2.3 Measurement

The following standardized questionnaires were used. To inventory the needs of persons with dementia, the Camberwell Assessment of Need for the Elderly (CANE) was used (interrater reliability: $r = 0.99$; test–retest reliability: $r = 0.96$) (Reynolds et al. 2000; Dröes et al. 2004). Background characteristics and context variables were collected with a standardized questionnaire administered by the carer. Cognitive functioning was assessed with the CAMCOG, a component of the Cambridge Examination for mental disorders in the elderly (Lindeboom et al. 1993) ($\alpha = 0.97$). Experienced Autonomy of persons with Dementia was assessed with the Experienced Autonomy list (Meiland and Dröes 2006) that was composed of seven items from the Mastery Scale (Pearlin and Schooler 1978) and five items that were adapted from the WHOQOL (WHO 2002); the quality of life in Alzheimer's Disease Scale (QoL-AD23, $\alpha = 0.88$–0.89).

The GP, specialist or programme coordinator of the meeting centres was contacted for information on the diagnosis of dementia and a clinical judgment about the severity of dementia with the Global Deterioration Scale (GDS (Reisberg et al. 1982)) (validity: $r = 0.53$–0.83).

6.2.4 Procedure

Workshops guidelines containing a checklist with the general workshop structure and the questions to be addressed were set up in advance and applied at all test sites. To structure the workshops and to stimulate the discussion, two PowerPoint presentations were used. One showed pictures of daily life situations and activities during the day. For each part of the day, it was discussed what activities persons with dementia performed, what they considered important for their quality of life, how this could be improved, and whether they experienced any problems or needs during specific parts of the day and/or with regard to specific activities in the four COGKNOW needs areas. All problems and needs mentioned in the four areas were listed on a flip chart and the participants were asked to prioritize them. The second PowerPoint presentation showed some examples of ICT solutions that have been developed for people with cognitive disabilities, or with dementia, in the four COGKNOW areas (e.g. electronic calendars and pictophone). These examples were used to stimulate the participants' own ideas and the discussion on preferences of ICT solutions for the inventoried needs in the selected needs areas. Both the workshop guidelines and the PowerPoint presentations were based on previous field and literature research on needs of people with dementia (Roest et al. 2007; Dröes et al. 2005) and assistive technology in dementia (Lauriks et al. 2007). In cases where participants could not, or did not, want to join the group workshops, individual interviews were conducted based on the same structure and content as the workshops. Participants initially received detailed information explaining the purpose and aim of the project. If they were willing to join, they were further involved in an informed consent procedure in which they were invited to participate in one project cycle of about 9 months. At the beginning of the workshops or individual interviews, all participants again confirmed their informed consent.

In Amsterdam, workshops were held at the memory clinic of the VU University Medical Centre and led by a senior researcher (psychologist), while a junior researcher (also a psychologist) took minutes. The workshops were audiotaped and a detailed report on the workshops was written up afterwards. The two workshops (one with the persons with dementia and one with the carers) both lasted approximately 3 h. Every participant received a summary of the workshop minutes afterwards. Because one couple had been on vacation during the time of the workshops, they were interviewed individually at home about their needs and preferred ICT solutions. In Belfast, the interviews were conducted by two trained dementia research nurses, who interviewed all patient–carer dyads individually at their homes and made written records. In Sweden, an assistant professor in social informatics carried out two group interviews and three individual interviews at the participants' homes (at this site data were also recorded in the form of written notes).

After the inventory of needs and preferred ICT solutions, individual interviews were carried out at the homes of the participants, where data were collected by means of the standardized scales.

At the beginning of the project researchers and other project members directly involved with participants were specifically trained in communication skills, ethics, data storage and privacy. All collected data were anonymized, individually coded and stored in computerized databases at the three research test sites. The key of the codes was kept in locked safety cabinets. Only anonymized data were exchanged between research sites.

6.2.5 Analysis

All research sites performed a descriptive analysis on background characteristics, cognitive (dis)abilities, context information, needs, experienced autonomy and quality of life of people with dementia, collected with the standardized questionnaires.

Detailed written reports were made of the audio recordings of the workshops and workshop interviews. A content analysis was done at each site to assess the most important needs and the most preferred ICT solutions in each of the four COGKNOW areas. Persons with dementia and carers were asked to state these priorities during the workshops. If there was no agreement on specific needs during the workshops, the most frequently (and strongly) mentioned needs were selected as having priority. The same method was used with regard to preferred ICT solutions. Two researchers at each site performed this analysis independently, and any discrepancies in the priority list were discussed until agreement was reached. Subsequently a top four list was made for the most appropriate solutions for the prioritized needs of the participants in the following way: (a) the ICT solution had to (at least partly) solve the prioritized need, (b) the ICT solutions that were preferred by the users were given preference and (c) existing ICT solutions that were previously tested on persons with dementia and had been proven helpful for them were given preference. Regarding this latter consideration, a literature review on ICT solutions was studied by all researchers (Lauriks et al. 2007).

Additionally, content analysis on the workshop and interview reports in Amsterdam was subject to an exploratory analysis, based on three theoretical frameworks that offer different conceptualizations of individual needs: the theory of 16 Basic Desires by Reiss (Reiss 2004), a model depicting basic needs and desires of people in general, needs described in the Netherlands National Dementia Programme (NDP) as related to problems that people with dementia generally encounter during the dementia process (Meerveld et al. 2004) and quality of life related needs of people with dementia (Dröes et al. 2006).

After that, possible scenarios were created (likely situations that the final COGKNOW ICT solution ultimately hopes to realize). The scenarios were based on the collected workshop and interview data and the top four lists from each research site. All three top four lists were then discussed with the technological partners in the project consortium to check on aspects of developmental feasibility. This resulted in a joint agreement on one overall top four list of devices or functionalities to be developed and tested in a first field test in which the emphasis would be on user-friendliness and usefulness of the ICT solution to be developed.

Finally, the information collected on background characteristics, cognitive (dis)abilities, context information, needs, experienced autonomy and wishes of people with dementia was used to specify the functional requirements for the agreed ICT solutions (Hettinga et al. 2007).

Table 6.1 depicts the different types of input on which was decided what functionalities to develop for the first field test.

Table 6.1 Types of input
used to decide on what to test
in field test #1 of the
COGKNOW project

Input types
User priority
Technical feasibility
Decision on which aspects are evaluated in field test
Scenarios
Strategic issues, project goals
Decision on what to test in field test

6.3 Results

6.3.1 Sample Characteristics

A total of 17 patient–carer dyads participated in the three test sites. Table 6.2 shows an overview of the participants' characteristics per site.

The persons with dementia varied in age from 56 to 86 years and except for one person in Amsterdam and two people in Belfast, all lived together with their main carer. Twelve out of seventeen people with dementia were limited in their mobility, either due to a physical complaint or due to spatial disorientation in unfamiliar surroundings. Several people with dementia at the three test sites suffered from medical complaints such as arthritis (four people), diabetes (two people) or hypertension (three people). Despite mobility constraints and medical complaints, none of the participants had installed safety measures in their homes yet.

6.3.2 Met and Unmet Needs and Wishes of Persons with Dementia

Descriptive analysis of all data on needs and wishes resulted in a detailed overview per site of met and unmet needs and wishes of people with dementia. Results of the needs inventory workshops and individual interviews were described for the four COGKNOW areas at each site. The overall results were analysed using three theoretical frameworks: first, Reiss's 16 Motives, which describe basic needs and desires of people in general (Reiss 2004); second, the NDP, which describes the specific needs related to problems people with dementia encounter (Meerveld et al. 2004); and third, the quality of life (QOL) domains, which describe needs regarding the quality of life of people with dementia (Dröes et al. 2006).

Table 6.3 gives an overview of the needs of people with dementia per COGKNOW area and the related descriptions of the three different theoretical frameworks.

6.3.2.1 Support for Memory

At all research sites, the predominant need in this area mentioned by people with dementia and their carers was the need to support their forgetfulness. People reported various problems with remembering, such as to take their medicine, to

Table 6.2 Characteristics of participants in the study

	Amsterdam ($n = 6$)	Belfast ($n = 6$)	Luleå ($n = 5$)
Persons with dementia			
Age (mean, range)	64,0 (56–78)	72,7 (65–86)	67,8 (60–77)
Sex			
Female	3	5	3
Male	3	1	2
Civil status			
Married	5	3	5
Divorced/widowed/single	1	3	–
Living alone	1	2	–
Cognitive disabilities			
GDS (mean, range)	3 (2–5)	3 (1–4)	3 (3–4)
Time orientation[a]	3	3	3
Place orientation[a]	0	0	1
Comprehension[a]	3	2	0
Reading comprehension[a]	0	0	0
Expression name[a]	4	0	2
Expression repeat[a]	4	5	2
Praxis[a]	2	5	0
Perception[a]	4	NA	0
Difficulty performing everyday activities[b]	3	2	1
Difficulty with mobility[b]	3	5	4
Carers			
Age (mean, range)	58,5 (49–78)	53,0 (40–72)	61,4 (23–78)
Sex			
Female	4	3	2
Male	2	3	3
Relation to patient			
Spouse	5	3	4
Child	1	2	1
Other (cousin)	–	1	–

[a]Results on the CAMCOG indicate problems with this cognitive function, in Lulea the CAMCOG was administered to only 4 persons
[b]Item of the experienced autonomy list
GDS = Global Deterioration Scale

take along their keys or phones when leaving the house, to know where they had put items, to remember their pin codes, appointments and the day or date. They expressed a great desire to compensate for this memory loss. People with dementia also described forgetfulness when it came to switching off electric appliances, how to cook or how to carry out household activities. Some people with dementia also had a need to be supported in remembering what was being said or what had happened recently. The carers confirmed these memory problems, adding that the need to be reminded to close doors or switch off electric appliances was of great priority. Across all research sites carers were concerned about the potential danger of this problem for their partners and themselves.

Table 6.3 Inventoried needs in the four COGKNOW areas during workshops and individual interviews and their relation to needs mentioned in three theoretical frameworks

COGKNOW area	Inventoried needs	Reiss's 16 motives	NDP	QoL
Memory	Need for being reminded of activities, appointments, location of items, pin codes closing and/or switching off devices/doors, personal hygiene, episodes of past (short and long term)	Independence Order Curiosity Tranquillity	What is the problem and what can help Physical care Danger Medical problems	Self-esteem/self-image Physical and mental health
Social contacts	Need for support with conversations, using phone, maintaining social contact	Status Social contact Acceptance	Avoiding contacts	Self-esteem/self-image Social contact Being useful/giving meaning to life
Daily activities	Need for support with finances, groceries, activities, hobbies	Independence Physical exercise Order Eating	Danger Loss	Enjoyment of activities Being useful/giving meaning to life Finances Self-determination and freedom
Feelings of safety	Need for security and safety cookers, turning-on/off devices, closing/locking doors, finances, being alone	Independence Tranquillity	Frightened, angry and confused Danger Loss	Attachment Finances Security + privacy Self-determination + freedom

6.3.2.2 Support for Social Contacts

The most important need, people with dementia in Amsterdam and Luleå voiced was the need to be supported in holding a conversation. Their word-finding and comprehension problems impeded initiating or maintaining conversations, either via the telephone or face to face, and made maintenance of social contacts difficult. Another difficulty, exacerbating social interaction, was the growing inability to use the phone, and consequently many had given up calling family or friends. In Belfast, people with dementia did report word-finding or comprehension difficulties as hindrance to social exchanges less frequently, but more frequently reported their forgetfulness of appointments, birthdays or names and expressed a need to be reminded in these areas.

Carers at all research sites agreed with these needs, but in Amsterdam and Lulea they explicitly reported another social problem that was not due to the inherent disabilities caused by Alzheimer's disease: the stigma associated with dementia had led former acquaintances or friends to withdraw. While carers could understand this in a way, at the same time they wished for more (public) openness regarding the diagnosis and course of the illness so that others would feel less intimidated by it.

6.3.2.3 Support for Daily Activities

At all test sites, people with dementia reported a great need for support in carrying out daily activities more independently. In line with the degree of progression of dementia, people differed in their perceived and reported difficulty to perform daily living activities. To help participants perform activities, automatic reminders could be useful. However, the majority of the participants commented they needed support not only to initiate an activity but also to carry on with it, expressing the need of step-wise assistance during the performance of activities. Activities they wanted support for ranged from household chores such as doing laundry, groceries and cooking or handling financial issues to pleasurable activities such as watching the TV or listening to the radio and to hobbies such as handcrafting, drawing, dancing, reading or parlour games. Across the three research sites different priority was given to the activities people with dementia wanted support for. While people in Amsterdam and Lulea attached importance to support with carrying out pleasurable activities, people in Belfast set particular value on being supported in household chores and in being reminded of taking their medication on time.

While carers agreed with the need for support in understanding written or oral instruction mentioned by their partners, they also reported a lack of initiative that they felt was even more to blame for the difficulties with daily activities. Disorientation in time and space caused further need for support in carrying out activities.

Beyond the abovementioned needs, people with dementia voiced a need that was closely related to feelings of autonomy, namely the need to be able and allowed to drive their car. People with dementia at all sites talked about the tremendous loss of independence they associated with having had to give up driving their cars.

While they understood the inevitability of giving up driving, they still mourned the resulting restriction to their mobility.

6.3.2.4 Feelings of Safety

The need to feel safe emerged forcefully in the participants' accounts of perceived insecurity in daily live. Forgetfulness, uncertainty about appropriate behaviour in demanding situations and difficulties carrying out daily activities caused insecurity and made people with dementia feel unsafe in their lives and in their homes. This was especially true of the dangers of forgetting to switch off electric appliances, or the gas cooker, having left the front door open or being unable to handle finances, and it concerned people with dementia at all research sites. Strikingly, people with dementia also felt they faced an enhanced risk of deception due to their weakness in remembering names or recognizing faces of people they met, either in public places or alone at home. Carers' accounts of needs in this area correspond with those of people with dementia. A meaningful way to indicate an emergency situation as well as being able to offer immediate help in case of emergency was a need that carers ascribed particular priority to.

6.3.3 Disabilities, Personal and Context Information Relevant for Developing ICT Solutions

Results from the interviews with persons with dementia and carers showed some dementia-related disabilities that were considered relevant for the development of an assistive technological device. These disabilities were memory and orientation problems; poor understanding of verbal instruction; difficulties with instrumental daily activities; and recognizing or understanding the meaning of pictures. Relevant personal and environmental features were persons with dementia living alone or with a carer; using aids like a cane; possessing technological appliances that were no longer easy to use; living in a house with multiple rooms and levels; and feeling insecure when being alone.

6.3.4 Final Top Four List

The decision on which ICT solutions would be developed in COGKNOW was based on the workshop and interview data outlined above, inventoried at each site and overall priorities of sites: to this end a table with priorities for ICT solutions was prepared per site (see Table 6.4) and this was discussed with the technical partners and the research site leaders, who also took into account the feasibility of developing the solutions within the project. This resulted in a final top four list of ICT solutions for the four COGKNOW areas.

Table 6.4 Top four list of preferred ICT solutions on the three test sites based on workshops with people with dementia and their carers and the literature on ICT solutions that have proven to be helpful for people with dementia

COGKNOW area of support focus	TOP4 Amsterdam	TOP4 Belfast	TOP4 Lulea	Conclusion on TOP4 for *first field test* after feasibility check with system designers
Support for memory Reminding and remembering	Reminder for not forgetting activities/appointments/take medicine. The solution should preferably be *stationary* with touch screen as well as *mobile*, e.g. Neuropage (Wilson et al. 2001; Hersh and Treadgold 1994)	Item locator, misplacement of items is a key early, and almost universal, symptom of a dementing illness – reflected in BCH workshops and literature review (see SMART home, BIME (Bath Institute of Medical Engineering)	Activity reminder/electronic calendar, stationary device with touch screen	*Reminding functionality +* locator mobile COGKNOW device *Examples in literature:* Neuropage, electronic calendar (ENABLE project: see also http://www.ihagen. no/english.htm http://www. enableproject.org/ html/products.html

Table 6.4 (continued)

COGKNOW area of support focus	TOP4 Amsterdam	TOP4 Belfast	TOP4 Lulea	Conclusion on TOP4 for *first field test* after feasibility check with system designers
Support for social contacts Enable communication with family and friends	Picture dialling function on touch screen integrated within the screen of the stationary device of the reminding system (thus not as a separate pictophone)	Electronic calendar with emphasis on appointments and social activities pending. Usefulness emphasized in workshops and within research community; see Forget-me-not http://www.ihagen.no/english.htm	Picture dialling function on touch screen integrated within the screen of the stationary device of the reminding system (thus not as a separate pictophone)	*Picture dialling functionality* *Examples in literature:* Photodialler (http://www.ellisenviro.com/news.html) Photophone (http://www.unisar.com/shoponline.asp?point=moreinfo &catid=&id=127) (http://www.enableproject.org/html/products.html) Photo contacts (mobile): (http://www.pocketx.net/smartphone/photocontacts.html)

Table 6.4 (continued)

COGKNOW area of support focus	TOP4 Amsterdam	TOP4 Belfast	TOP4 Lulea	Conclusion on TOP4 for *first field test* after feasibility check with system designers
Support with daily activities Help executing activities that provide pleasure, recreational activities, useful activities	Support for activities for pleasure, e.g. picture gramophone ENABLE project (Adlam et al. 2004) integrated within touch screen of activity reminder or picture of TV on touch screen that starts the TV when touched	Pill dispenser – medication management issue identified as an important "daily activity" particularly within workshops and concerning elderly persons generally	Support for activities for pleasure, e.g. picture of TV on touch screen of the stationary device of the activity reminder that starts the TV when touched	*Support functionality* for activities for pleasure on stationary device with touch screen to turn on, e.g. radio/TV media playback *Examples in literature*: picture gramophone (ENABLE project: http://www.enableproject.org/html/products.html

Table 6.4 (continued)

COGKNOW area of support focus	TOP4 Amsterdam	TOP4 Belfast	TOP4 Lulea	Conclusion on TOP4 for *first field test* after feasibility check with system designers
Enhance feelings of safety Prevent people with dementia from experiencing anxious or dangerous situations	Support during cooking, e.g. cooker usage monitor ENABLE project (Adlam et al. 2004). Signal on stationary and mobile activity reminder device or Warning to close door/take things outdoors such as keys or simple mobile phone with or without GPS, e.g. Mobile Coach (Kort 2005)	Picture telephone identified in workshop discussions and see Mobile Telecoach (Kort 2005)	Reminder to turn devices of on stationary device, for example, the stove (not as a separate artefact, but as a function within the activity reminder system) or Direct or easy contact possibilities to a service or emergency line (not as a separate artefact, but as a function within the reminder system)	Warning to close and/or lock front door Reminder to take mobile phone outside Easy emergency contact

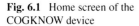 **Fig. 6.1** Home screen of the COGKNOW device

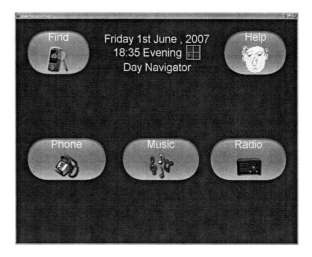

It was decided to develop a stationary component, such as a tablet PC with touch screen, and a mobile component featuring the same functions as the stationary component but allowing the person with dementia to make and receive phone calls outdoors as well. Only simple written instructions were to be used on the devices (the cohort's language deficits recorded on the CAMCOG showed that almost one-third of the participants had problems with verbal instructions). See Fig. 6.1 for a screenshot of the touch screen.

For the area "support for memory" it was decided to realize a reminding service to provide prompts to help people remember to eat meals, make phone calls and carry out personal hygiene such as brushing their teeth. Also, the day and date would be featured on the devices to support people with orientation in time. Additionally, the ICT device would contain a function that locates the mobile phone component in case the person with dementia has misplaced it.

Excerpts of one of the two scenarios, which were developed during the analyses, show a reminder service to be developed and tested in Field Test 1. It is used by a woman with dementia, who lives together with her husband.

> When Anne was diagnosed with Alzheimer's disease, her husband Jim had the COGKNOW day navigator system installed, to help them both through the day. The COGKNOW day navigator is a tablet PC that also includes a separate mobile device, which can be used in and outside the house. The COGKNOW day navigator can be configured according to the particular needs of each person. Jim and Anne decided together on which reminders they considered as supporting for Anne, and Jim could easily program the chosen reminders, such as reminding Anne to eat her meals or brush her teeth as she often forgets these activities.

For the area "support for social contact", a picture dialling function was agreed upon to facilitate making or receiving phone calls. The picture dialling service aims to support the person with dementia in calling a person by simply pressing on his or her picture, either on the stationary device or on the mobile device, without having to remember or dial any phone number. In the following excerpt of a scenario, the use of the picture dialling function is illustrated:

> Jim had inserted photographs of their children in the COGKNOW day navigator so that Anne could phone them easily by touching the screen when she felt alone or insecure in the absence of her husband. She is then quickly connected and if her daughter cannot answer the phone, Anne can easily contact another person using the picture dialling contact list.

To support people with dementia with "daily activities" it was decided to develop an entertainment service in the form of a radio control and music player. It enables people with dementia to engage in pleasurable activities, such as listening to music or to the radio, which they cannot carry out on their own anymore, because they have difficulty operating devices. Again, an excerpt of the developed scenarios, in this case a 74-year-old widower living alone.

> The COGKNOW day navigator asks Martin whether he wants to listen to the music or the radio. Martin decides to listen to the radio and presses the radio picture on the touch screen of the tablet PC. For music, he simply has to touch the music notes symbol and previously programmed music pieces are replayed. In case he is not content with the music piece that the system plays, all Martin has to do is double click on the music notes picture and the next song is played.

For the final area, "enhance feelings of safety", a warning service that would detect open or closed doors was agreed upon. Additionally, it was decided to install an emergency call function in the system so that the person with dementia would be able to call for help easily. The warning service should offer audio and visual warnings, available on both the stationary and the mobile device.

In the following scenario excerpt about Martin, the male widower living alone, it is explained how the warning service and emergency function could be of help.

> Due to his forgetfulness, Martin frequently forgets to close his front door, which is then left open all day long and sometimes during the night as well. Since Martin has been using the COGKNOW navigator he is reminded to close the door in case he has forgotten to do so. The COGKNOW warning service alerts Martin with a beep to close the door. In case Martin falls or some other emergency situation occurs, Martin can easily call for help. By simply pressing the emergency button on the stationary or mobile device, the system automatically connects him with his son, the agreed primary contact in case of emergency. If his son is not available, the system automatically connects Martin with another contact.

6.4 Discussion and Conclusion

This chapter describes the development process of an ICT solution aimed to help persons with dementia experience more autonomy and an enhanced quality of life. Right from the start of the COGKNOW project, persons with dementia and their carers were involved in the developmental process that consists of three iterations in which user needs are assessed and consequently discussed among clinical dementia experts and technological system designers to ensure a good translation of needs into functional requirements and design specifications. This chapter focused on the first iteration of the study.

In the area of memory, persons with dementia preferred support with remembering daily activities, the locations of items and switching off devices in the home. In the area of social contact, people wished to be supported in maintaining contact with their social network. In the area of daily activities, people wanted to be supported in performing these activities more independently. The need to feel safe became apparent from persons with dementia reporting feelings of insecurity and uncertainty. Dangers resulting from forgetting to switch off appliances or close the door were particularly relevant to both persons with dementia and their carers.

People with dementia and carers preferred the following ICT solutions: reminders for activities, the time and an item locator; a simple solution for contacting family members such as a picture dialling phone; assistance with turning on music or television; and an automatic switch-off for devices.

Finally, taking into account the cognitive disabilities of the persons with dementia and the technical feasibility of developing solutions within the time frame of the project, it was decided that for the first prototype of the cognitive prosthetic ICT device the following would be developed: in the area of remembering – a day and time indication, a find mobile service and reminding service; in the area of social contact – a picture dialling function; in the area of daily activities – a media playback and radio function, and in the area of safety, a warning device for an open front door and an emergency service. The preferred ICT solutions inventoried in the study correspond partly with other studies among persons with dementia, e.g. Sixsmith (Sixmith et al. 2007a, 2007b) who proposed technological devices such as a simple music player and a photo phone and Wherton (Wherton and Monk 2008) who recommended technological support for leisure activities, communication and enhancing safety.

In discussing and describing the needs, we found that the frameworks of the NDP25 and the quality of life domains (Dröes et al. 2006) helped to make the perceived needs more concrete in the daily life of persons with dementia and carers. A more general description of needs of persons was found in the theory of Reiss on motives and desires (Reiss 2004). Not all motives, domains of quality of life and problem areas were reflected in the needs and wants expressed in this study. This was partly caused by the selective focus in the COGKNOW project on four need areas and partly because only persons with mild dementia were recruited for participation in the project.

Although the study was set up carefully, there were some limitations. First of all, the needs assessment was conducted among groups of people with dementia and informal carers in three Northern European countries. People from other parts of Europe were not represented in the study sample. Therefore the study results are not necessarily valid for people with dementia living in other parts of Europe. Second, we tried to compose a varied group by randomly recruiting persons with dementia and carers who differed in characteristics that might be related to needs, e.g. age, gender, living alone or not, type of relationship between person with dementia and carer and rural or non-rural living area. Nevertheless, the majority of the recruited persons with dementia were married and lived together with the carer. This may have caused an underrepresentation of needs and wishes experienced by persons with dementia who live alone. Finally, some persons in the very early stages of dementia felt they did not need support yet. On the other hand, these persons were able to articulate clearly what they found important in their daily life and imagine what might be useful to them in the future. Our experiences in this study reflect the view that it is important to assess and understand in-depth the needs and wishes of persons with dementia and their preferences for ICT solutions. It helps to understand how to translate these needs into functional requirements when developing assistive technology for this target group. Besides that, to increase the chance of developing an ICT device that would be useful for persons with dementia in general, the COGKNOW project focused on four need areas that in a large-scale survey of one of the COGKNOW consortium partners were identified as frequently unmet in persons with dementia (van der Roest et al. 2009). Subsequently, the final plans for developing assistive technology in the COGKNOW need areas were based both on the results of the user workshops and interviews in our study, and on research findings regarding the use of assistive technology in dementia as described in the literature (Lauriks et al. 2007; Adlam et al. 2004; Nugent et al. 2005; Kort 2005).

As the development of an ICT product is a long and complex process, it is advisable to involve potential users in different phases of this process, to attune the ICT product as much as possible to the needs and wishes of the future users and to make it more user-friendly and useful. Within COGKNOW, the needs and wishes of the persons with dementia and carers are assessed in the start of the prototype development as well as in the later stages. Persons with dementia and carers were also directly involved in the evaluation of the prototype. The developmental method applied in COGKNOW is best typified as a user-participatory approach (Helander 2006), first because the four target areas chosen for development of the ICT device were based on findings from research on needs reported by persons with dementia themselves, second because the needs and potential ICT solutions were elaborated by interviewing potential end-users, and third because the prototype is also evaluated by end-users by means of field tests. The data collected among users will be used as input for the further development of the device. We aim to develop our ICT solution for people with mild dementia living in the community. However, it is anticipated that because of the variability even in people with mild dementia (e.g. in cognitive disabilities, mobility and living circumstances), ICT solutions need to be adaptable to needs and preferences of individual persons with dementia and their carers. These personalization aspects will be further explored in the project. In the final stage of the study the ICT solution will be evaluated on user-friendliness, usefulness and impact on autonomy and quality of life of the persons with dementia.

Besides the involvement of potential end-users, we also recommend a multidisciplinary team approach: only clinical researchers and technological system designers working together will be able to translate the needs of persons with dementia into functional requirements of assistive technology.

To conclude, both a user-participatory design and a multidisciplinary approach may help to develop more user-friendly and useful products for persons with dementia and their carers, that will gain easier acceptance by the target group. Acceptance is an important precondition for effectively integrating technological applications as an additional means of supporting people with dementia at home.

References

Adlam, T., Faulkner, R., Orpwood, R. et al. (2004) The installation and support of internationally distributed equipment for people with dementia. IEEE Transactions on Information Technology in Biomedicine, 8:253–257.
Andersson, N.B., Hanson, E., Magnusson, L. (2002) Views of family carers and older people of information technology. British Journal of Nursing, 11:827–831.
ASTRID (2000) ASTRID: A Guide to Using Technology Within Dementia Care. Hawker Publications, London.
Cohene, T., Baecker, R., Marziali, E. (2005) Designing Interactive Life Story Multimedia for a Family Affected by Alzheimer's Disease: A Case Study. CHI 2005, April 2–7, Portland Oregon, USA.
Dröes, R.M., Boelens, E.J., Bos, J. et al. (2006) Quality of life in dementia in perspective: An explorative study of variations in opinions among people with dementia and their professional caregivers, and in literature. Dementia: International Journal of Social Research and Practice, 5:533–558.
Dröes, R.M., Meiland, F.J.M., van der Roest, H.G. et al. (2005) Opportunities for We-Centric Service Bundling in Dementia Care. Freeband Frux Projectpartners, Amsterdam.
Dröes, R.M., van Hout, H.P.J., van der Ploeg, E.S. (2004) Camberwell Assessment of Need for the Elderly (CANE), Revised Version (IV). VU Free University Medical Hospital, Department of Psychiatry, EMGO Institute, Amsterdam.
Ferri, C.P., Prince, M., Brayne, C. et al. (2005) Global prevalence of dementia: A Delphi consensus study. Lancet, 366:2112–2117.
Gaugler, J.E., Kane, R.L., Kane, R.A. et al. (2005) Unmet care needs and key outcomes in dementia. JAGS, 53:2098–2105.
Hagen, I., Holthe, T., Duff, P. et al (2002) A systematic assessment of assistive technology. Journal of Dementia Care, 10:26–28.
Health Council Netherlands. (2002) Dementia. Health Council of the Netherlands, The Hague.
Helander, M. (2006) A Guide to Human Factors and Ergnomics, 2nd edn. Taylor & Francis group, UK.
Hersh, N., Treadgold, L. (1994) Rehabilitation of memory dysfunction by prosthetic memory & cueing. Neurorehabilitation, 4(3):187–197.
Hettinga, M., Andersson, A.L., Dröes, R.M. et al. (2007) COGKNOW Project, Deliverable 1.4.1. Functional Requirements Specification. COGKNOW Consortium.
Kort, S. (2005) Mobile Coaching. A pilot study into the user-friendliness and effects of Mobile Coaching on the wellbeing of people with dementia and their informal caregivers. MSc thesis, Faculty of Psychology, Vrije Universiteit, Amsterdam.
Lauriks, S., Reinersmann, A., van der Roest, H.G . et al. (2007). Review of ICT-based services for identified unmet needs in people with dementia. Ageing Research Reviews, 6: 223–246.
Lindeboom, J., Ter Horst, R., Hooyer, C. et al. (1993) Some psychometric properties of the CAMCOG. Psychological Medicine, 23:213–219.
Meerveld, J., Schumacher, J., Krijger, E. et al. (2004) Landelijk Dementieprogramma, werkboek. NIZW, Utrecht.
Meiland, F.J.M., Dröes, R.M. (2006) Experienced Autonomy. VU Free University Medical Hospital, Department of Psychiatry, EMGO Institute, Amsterdam.
Nugent, C.D. (2007) ICT in the elderly and dementia [Editorial]. Aging and Mental Health, 11(5):473–476.

Nugent, C., Finlay, D., Davies, R. et al. (2005) Can technology improve compliance to medica-tion? In: S. Giroux, H. Pigot (eds.) From Smart Homes to Smart Care. IOS press, Amsterdam, pp. 65–72.

Nygard, L., Starkhammar, S. (2007) The use of everyday technology by people with dementia living alone: Mapping out the difficulties. Aging and Mental Health, 11:144–155.

Orpwood, R., Gibbs, C., Adlam, T. et al. (2005) The design of smart homes for people with dementia: User interface aspects. Universal Access in the Information Society, 4:156–164.

Pearlin, L.I., Schooler, C. (1978) The structure of coping. Journal of Health and Social Behavior, 19:2–21.

Reisberg, B., Ferris, S., De Leon, M.J. et al. (1982) The global deterioration scale for assessment of primary degenerative dementia. The American Journal of Psychiatry, 139:1136–1139.

Reiss, S. (2004) Multifaceted nature of intrinsic motivation: The theory of 16 basic desires. Review of General Psychology, 8:179–193.

Reynolds, T., Thornicroft, G., Abas, M. et al. (2000) Camberwell Assessment of Need for the Elderly (CANE): Development, validity and reliability. British Journal of Psychiatry, 176: 444–452.

Sixsmith, A.J., Gibson, G., Orpwood, R.D. et al. (2007a) Developing a technology 'wish-list' to enhance the quality of life of people with dementia. Gerontechnology, 6:2–19.

Sixsmith, A., Orpwood, R., Torrington, J. (2007b) Quality of life technologies for people with dementia: Topics in geriatric rehabilitation. Smart Technology, 23:85–93.

van der Roest, H.G., Meiland, F.J.M., Comijs, H.C. et al. (2009) What do community-dwelling people with dementia need? A survey among those who are known to care and welfare services. International Psychogeriatrics, 21(5): 949–965.

van der Roest, H.G., Meiland, F.J.M., Maroccini, R. et al. (2007) Subjective needs of people with dementia: A review of the literature. International Psychogeriatrics, 19:559–592.

WHO SRPB Quality of Life Group. (2002) WHOQOL-SRPB Field Test Instrument. Department of Mental Health & Substance Dependence, WHO, Geneva, Switzerland.

Wherton, J.P., Monk, A.F. 2008. Technological opportunities for supporting people with dementia who are living at home. International Journal of Human-Computer Studies, 571–586.

Wilson, B.A., Emslie, H.C., Quirk, K., Evans, J.J. (April 2001) Reducing everyday memory and planning problems by means of a paging system: A randomised control crossover study. Journal of Neurology and Neurosurgery and Psychiatry, 70(4):477–482.

Chapter 7
Managing the Transition from User Studies to Functional Requirements to Technical Specification

Marike Hettinga, Chris D. Nugent, Richard Davies, Ferial Moelaert, Halgeir Holthe, and Anna-Lena Andersson

Abstract In this chapter the management of the process that bridges the large step between user studies and the design of the system is described. This process consists of two substeps: the transition from user requirements to functional requirements and from the latter to the technical specification. The chapter begins by describing the concepts of functional requirements and technical specifications. Following this the two subprocesses are described and the lessons that are learned are outlined. At the end of the chapter the work carried out is summarised using a list of recommendations for future design projects that may be of a similar nature within this domain.

7.1 Introduction

The prevailing perception on the role and contribution of, on the one hand, social scientists and, on the other hand, technical scientists in user-centred design and development projects is sometimes limited to an image of two separate processes that are carried out successively in time. The first process of gathering user data, needs, desires and abilities of the target group, is followed by the second process of technical design and development of the applications based on the information elicited from the first stage. Such a distinction between the two subprocesses is not advisable. It is important to appreciate that the role of the social scientists, does not end after user studies have been performed and technical persons are informed about the desires. Similarly, it is important to appreciate that the role of technical scientists does not necessarily only begin after the handing over of the functional requirements (FRs).

M. Hettinga (✉)
Novay, Enschede, The Netherlands
e-mail: marike.hettinga@novay.nl

M.D. Mulvenna, C.D. Nugent (eds.), *Supporting People with Dementia Using Pervasive Health Technologies*, Advanced Information and Knowledge Processing, DOI 10.1007/978-1-84882-551-2_7, © Springer-Verlag London Limited 2010

After gathering the user data a critical step needs to be undertaken: the transition from user data to FRs and following this to the technical specification (TS). This transition cannot be performed without the support of both social and technical scientists.

In this chapter we explain why it is of such importance to have all disciplines involved in the transition phase. To illustrate this position we use both positive experiences and learning experiences of the transition process in the COGKNOW project and demonstrate how within our work we have progressed from the user requirements (UR) to the TS. We conclude this chapter with recommendations that we hope to be of use for future design projects.

7.2 Explaining the Concepts of FRs and TS

FRs form the bridge between the URs on the one hand and the TS on the other. The URs can be viewed as the result of the user studies, while the TS is used as input for the design and development of the desired applications. This process is depicted in Fig. 7.1.

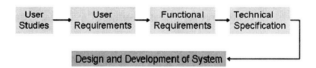

Fig. 7.1 The process from user requirements to design and development

Before discussing the process of moving from URs to the TS in the following sections, we explain these concepts further by means of an example.

Consider the situation where the user studies reveal that users often stress the following: "If you remind me once what I have to do, I will forget. It has to be repeated a few times."

The corresponding FR could then be formulated as a desire of some system or service to provide a "repetition of reminder". Based on this, the FR requires a detailed specification before it can be integrated in the TS. To produce this level of detail will require answering questions such as "how often does it need to be repeated", "with which time interval should the repetition occur", "does this interval need to decrease", to name but a few. After answering all these questions, it then becomes possible to cncapsulate all of this information within the TS, as depicted in Fig. 7.2.

This example is taken from one of the slideshows presented during a meeting with all project members. It was experienced within the COGKNOW project that abstract concepts like FRs and TS were difficult to grasp for people with a non-technical background. It was also found that the importance of the FRs and TS was not clear to such a group.

FRs are extremely important because they represent the information elicited from the users in the initial user studies in addition to specifying all functionalities that

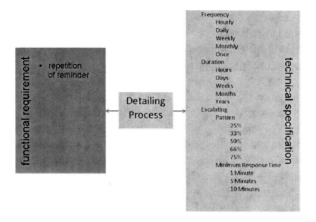

Fig. 7.2 An example of an FR and the corresponding TS

may be developed during the project. Hence, they can be viewed as forming one of the core elements of a user-centred design project whereby it becomes possible to state that all user study results are reflected within the FRs.

After each field test in the COGKNOW project, which gave new user feedback, the FRs were evaluated and adjusted, giving new input to the TS. This central role was underestimated in the beginning of the project as was the process to deliver the FRs.

For those viewing the process as depicted in 7.1 for the first time, namely translating URs to FRs to TS, this may evoke the image of a straightforward, almost mathematical process. Nothing is further from the truth. The key to this process is all about reaching a common understanding in relation to what is going to be developed and how this function will be realised in a tangible entity. Reaching this common understanding is a delicate and complex process in which user study results are balanced against technical feasibilities and project time constraints and resources (both financial and man power). Accomplishing this process successfully, both from a process and output perspective, will establish robust foundations for the remainder of a project. With the well-known delays and other setbacks of IT-development projects, such a foundation is well needed.

7.3 From URs to FRs: Reaching a Common Understanding

The questions to be asked at this stage in the process include

- How to start with formulating FRs after analysing the user data?
- Which functionalities do we wish to include?
- Which level of detail should be specified?
- Which additional information should be included for each explicit FR?

Many questions, combined with the lacking sense of importance of the FRs can quickly lead to postponement of the first iteration of the set of FRs. The overwhelming amount of information stemming from the user studies can make project members hesitant to start formulating the first concrete set of FRs. Indeed, in some instances it may be perceived that formulating FRs results in abstracting away from the user needs and conditions.

Hence, a key issue is therefore to ensure that such an impasse is overcome. Within our current work, in the first instance, motivation was experienced from a movie that was created using the preliminary results of the user studies (see http://cogknow.eu/). This movie conveyed the concept of a person with dementia in his own house engaging in several everyday situations in which he was supported by an ICT application. This movie served within the project as a frame of reference. By means of using "natural language" project members from all disciplines were able to discuss features of the proposed application while referring to situations in the movie. The movie provided them with a common understanding of possible functionalities and how these functionalities could be used in daily practice.

In the COGKNOW project this frame of reference served, together with the user results, as input for an initial version of the FRs. This version was developed by two researchers: one with a background in social sciences and one with a technical background.

The initial version of the FRs acted as a discussion medium. Their delivery suddenly aroused the attention of many project members. Discussions about the content of the set of FRs, their format, the structure, the information which was included and many other related topics were raised. These discussions turned out to be very fruitful: many decisions were made that had their impact on the future years of the project. An important element of these discussions was that they included researchers from all disciplines.

7.4 Completing the FRs

In the previous section we described the process that led to the initial version of the FRs. In this section we describe the process adopted to obtain a complete list of FRs. This process was highly iterative and conducted by a small team within the project. The FR team ($n = 5$), was comprised of both technical, social and clinical scientists. The team adopted a four-step cycle, using the initial set of the FRs as a starting point. The process which was adopted involved the following process:

1. Mapping the FRs to the TS.
2. Based on the outcomes of the above step, adjust the FRs, level of detail, consistency, clarity, structure, etc.
3. Add references in the user study results referring to specific FRs.
4. Check the FRs with the results from the user studies to ensure completeness.

The above cycle was iterated until a satisfactory set of FRs was produced. This moment was reached when the involved social scientists indicated that all user study results were integrated in the FRs and the technical scientists were content with the level of detail: the FRs provided a sufficient amount of information for them to build on.

The final step towards a fully completed list of FRs involved extending the FRs document to a broader group in order to attain a complete consensus among the project consortium. This final check was considered to be essential given the importance being placed on the FRs as the primary bridge between user needs and the technical prototypes which were to be developed.

Following completion of the above process, during a face-to-face project meeting, four groups were formed with each group being assigned to one of the four main categories of the COGKNOW Project: remembering, communication, activities of pleasure, and safety; see previous chapters within this book for more details on these categories. Groups comprising of between seven to eight people were formed to ensure that they offered a balance in expertise between clinical and technical personnel. The primary task for each group was to examine the FR document for completeness and detail. Additional tasks bestowed upon each group were to further refine which FRs would be considered for development during the first iteration of the project. This was performed by considering the technical feasibility, project vision and the top four functionalities as reported by the user workshops across all three test sites; see previous chapters within this book for more information on the selected functionalities per field test. These discussions took place within the four groups during a series of face-to-face meetings which were held over a period of 2 days.

7.4.1 Presentation of the FRs

The FRs were separated into four lists with each list representing one of the main COGKNOW areas as discussed in the above. Both functional and non-functional requirements were included as distinguishing between them was not always feasible. The labels shown in Table 7.1 provide an overview of the information used to describe each individual FR.

An example of a number of FRs is presented in Fig. 7.3. In this instance only the most important labels have been included.

In line with the example shown in Fig. 7.3 four lists of FRs were provided to the technical scientists in the project.

7.5 Translating the FRs to Technical Specs

Once the FRs were established and documented in a manner agreeable by all within the project the level of detail captured was subsequently translated to the TS. There are a number of approaches which may be adopted to translate the FRs to the TS. The approach adopted within the COGKNOW project was largely based on the use

Table 7.1 The labels describing each FR

ID	This is a unique four digit number. Once a FR is identified with a number, this number will not be changed or deleted anymore
Title	Short title for easy referencing. First-level requirements are in bold
Description	Detailed description of the FR
Priority	Each of the three test sites indicated which priority their users gave to this FR with the following levels: low: users do not think it is relevant medium: one or some people mention(s) it/they think it might be relevant in the future high: people gave this priority themselves or 3 or more people mentioned it or 1 (or more) strongly expressed this need
Technical feasibility	Provides an indication if FR can be realised from a technical development perspective taking into account project constraints of time and available resources (man power and budget)
Trial number	Provides an indication of which field trial (1, 2 or 3) FR will be realised for
Source	Refers to the source from which the requirement is derived. For example, workshops, interviews, literature. References to specific user study reports are also included
Rationale	Explains why this requirement is needed
Dependency	Indicates whether there are dependencies with other requirements
Author	Indicates who added the requirement to the list. This allows others to ask for further explanation of this requirement
Comments	Any notes or remarks about the requirement

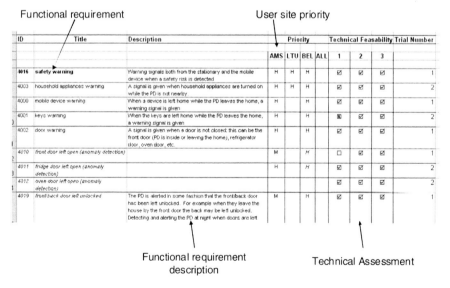

Fig. 7.3 An example of a few FRs and their labels

of use cases. It was felt that within such a multidisciplinary team the readability of the TS would be enhanced if such an approach were to be adopted.

As previously mentioned, following the ranking of the FRs, the first iteration of the project focused on the presentation of material which addressed the priority issues across the four main areas of the project. In terms of documenting the TS was presented in four main sections, one for each of the four areas. In addition, to assist with the volume of documentation two complimentary TS were developed. The first TS addressed the mobile component of the system and its interaction with the home environment. The second TS addressed the server component of the system and how it interacted with, stored and managed data which were collected from the home environment.

The approach which was adopted to translate the FRs to the TS was as follows:

Title of TS element	This was the title given to the element within the TS which could be mapped directly onto the corresponding FR
Description	This provides a detailed description in a natural language of the exact function alities which will be undertaken
Prerequisites	This provides the details of any actions which may occur and have an impact on the functionality/service which is being described
Use case/steps	The exact details of the step to each functionality are presented
Sequence diagram	A visual representation in the form of a sequence diagram is used to convey the process of information and control flow between each entity

Figures 7.4 and 7.5 show examples of the aforementioned structure which were developed as part of the TS for the COGKNOW project.

In addition to providing low-level technical details which explain each of the FRs in a technical sense it is also a requirement of the TS to provide a logical overview of the system architecture which is to be implemented. A logical view of the system architecture provides a description of the main components within the system, their organisation and linkages/workflow with subsystems.

Other components of the TS which are required to support realisation of the systems included

- database schema
- protocol for message passing along with message structure
- rendering of data for user interfaces

To further complement the presentation of this information, details of operating platforms, products and communication networks should also be taken into

3.1.2.2.   Picture dialling via CHH hands-free system

Description

This use case describes the placement of a phone call by the PD via touching a picture of the requested contact via the touch screen.

The call is initiated by touching the picture of the intended recipient via the touch screen. Initially the PD will be presented with a menu or home screen that will contain an icon or an image that represents the picture dialling service. Once selected the PD will be presented will the picture dialling service, which will consist of a contact picture list. The PD performs the phone call via the CHH hands-free system.

The underlying backbone of this service will be PSTN. A traditional phone interface will be used to facilitate any communication. Selecting a contact will automatically dial and connect the call to the requested party. All interactions are sent to the server for logging.

Prerequisites:

- None

Steps:

Step number	Step description
1	The PD selects the request contact via the GUI by scrolling a list of photos associated with the contacts. The PD finally chooses the person to be dialled by touching the associated picture.
2	The CCA establishes the call and provides a visual signal reinforced by a voice announcement when the call is active.
3	The PD speaks with the contact using the CHH hands-free system

Fig. 7.4 Excerpt from the COGKNOW TS showing the process used to represent components within the TS

consideration. Chapter 10 within this book provides further details of the realisation of the TS in terms of a COGKNOW prototype.

7.6 Recommendations

In the former sections of this chapter we described the process from user studies to technical specification. In this final section we present our lessons learned and formulate them as recommendations for future projects.

7.6.1 Common Understanding of Future System Use

Create a common understanding between all project members about the target group and the situations in which they will use the system and all its functionalities.

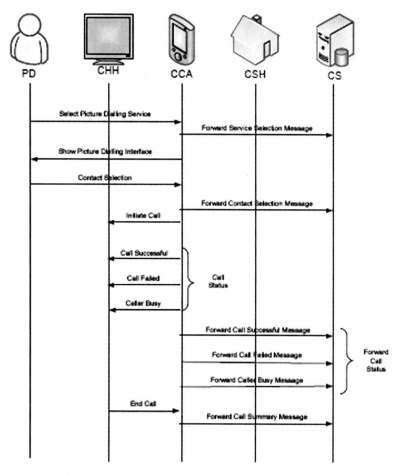

Fig. 7.5 Excerpt from the COGKNOW TS showing the process used to represent components within the TS

Especially in a multidisciplinary project (with the extra complication of multi-linguistic) a shared frame of reference in natural language is needed. In the COGKNOW project this frame of reference was provided by the COGKNOW movie. It can, however, also be rich case descriptions or scenarios of the situations in which a target group member needs (or receives) ICT support.

7.6.2 Abstract Technical Concepts

A first recommendation concerns the abstract technical concepts like FRs and TS are difficult to grasp for non-technical people. Use realistic examples early in the project to clarify the concepts of FRs and TS. Most optimal would be learning by doing: form small multidisciplinary groups of project members who take a UR and formulate the corresponding FRs and TS.

7.6.3 Central Role of FRs

Stress the central role of the FRs: the more this is clear to project members, the more they are motivated to participate in the process leading to the FRs. And, as argued above, participation of all disciplines in the project is important.

7.6.4 The Initial Version of FRs

Do not postpone formulating an initial version of the FRs. The initial version will stimulate fruitful discussions hence progressing work within the project. Postponing is a natural thing to do since the initial version of FRs requires the step from more broadly described functions to precisely defined requirements. Such a step is difficult to grasp.

7.6.5 More General: Vehicles for Communication Are Crucial

Vehicles for communication (like rich case descriptions, or FRs) are crucial to a project, especially for one with multidisciplinary and multi-linguistic project members. Create them as soon as possible and hence do not worry too much about the exact content or format: it is the discussion that follows which has the value.

7.6.6 One Coordinator for FRs

Designate one researcher with the coordination and responsibility of delivering the FRs. This person should provide the necessary vehicles for discussion. Obviously this researcher can rely on others for support.

7.6.7 Iterative Multidisciplinary Process to FRs

All disciplines involved in the project should also be involved in the process of delivering FRs. A successful way of proceeding is an iterative manner: adding more detail in each iteration between disciplines. The iterations between disciplines should also be visualised in the documents: in the FR lists cross-references between user study results and FRs should be included.

7.6.8 Translation Process of FRs to TS

The translation of mapping between the FRs and the TS should be coordinated by the designated researchers leading both respective processes. Finalisation of the process should only be deemed completed once several iterations of refinement have been undertaken to ensure both are in agreement with shared language and concepts being used.

Chapter 8
Dementia-Related and Other Factors to Be Taken into Account When Developing ICT Support for People with Dementia – Lessons from Field Trials

Rose-Marie Dröes, Sanne Bentvelzen, Franka Meiland, and David Craig

Abstract When developing assistive technology for people with dementia it is important to take into account their needs and wishes as well as their cognitive abilities and disabilities. In this chapter we describe how the disabilities accompanying dementia can be taken into account when developing assistive technological devices for this target group. As a case example, we used the COGKNOW project, which specifically focuses on developing ICT support for people with mild dementia in the areas of memory, social contact, daily activities and feelings of safety. Before device development in the first year of the project, workshops and interviews involving 17 persons with dementia and their carers were held to discuss their needs, wishes and disabilities and some background and environmental information were obtained. The main dementia-related disabilities that emerged from this cohort and that proved relevant for the development of an assistive technological device were memory and orientation problems, poor understanding of verbal instruction, difficulty with instrumental daily activities and recognizing/understanding the meaning of pictures. Relevant personal and environmental features were living alone or with a carer, the need for company and social contact, the need for support in doing things for fun, using aids like a walking cane, possessing technological appliances that could not be easily used anymore, living in a house with multiple rooms and levels and feeling insecure when being alone. Taken into account these disabilities, background and environmental features, functional requirements were specified and a device was developed, the COGKNOW Day Navigator Version 1 (CDNv-1). The aim of the CDN was to support people with dementia in reminding, social contact, daily activities and safety in a simple manner. After a development period, the user friendliness and usefulness of this device were assessed via a field test in which the CDNv-1 was tested with 16 people with mild dementia and their carers in their

R.-M. Dröes (✉)
Department of Psychiatry, Alzheimer Center (EMGO-Institute), VU University Medical Centre/Regional Institute for Mental Health Services GGZ-in Geest, Amsterdam, The Netherlands
e-mail: rm.droes@vumc.nl

M.D. Mulvenna, C.D. Nugent (eds.), *Supporting People with Dementia Using Pervasive Health Technologies*, Advanced Information and Knowledge Processing, DOI 10.1007/978-1-84882-551-2_8, © Springer-Verlag London Limited 2010

own home. By means of semi-structured interviews and observations, experiences of the persons with dementia and carers with the CDN were inventoried. It was concluded that though most functions were judged as user friendly and useful, further personalization of the CDN would improve the perceived user friendliness and usefulness. This study showed that detailed information on the person with dementia's functioning and living environment is necessary to attune assistive technology to their needs. The group of persons with dementia that participated in this project also showed that people with mild dementia are very capable of giving their opinion on the user friendliness and usefulness of assistive technology.

8.1 Introduction

When developing assistive technology for people with dementia it is important to take into account their needs and wishes as well as their cognitive abilities and disabilities (including the changes in behaviour that can accompany these disabilities) (ASTRID 2000; Orpwood et al. 2005; Sixsmith et al. 2007). In Chapter 4, a global overview of the cognitive impairments that occur in dementia, such as problems with language, executive functions and recognizing the meaning of objects, as well as of the disabilities that occur in daily life as a consequence of these impairments, was presented.

In this chapter we will describe how the disabilities accompanying dementia must be taken into account when developing assistive technological devices for people with dementia. We will use the COGKNOW project as a case example and will therefore focus specifically on people with *mild* dementia, as they are the target group of this project, and the four functional areas that COGKNOW aims to support, i.e. memory, social contact, activities in daily life and feelings of safety. We will base our descriptions on experiences and data gathered in the first year of the project in which a first version of the so-called COGKNOW Day Navigator (CDN) was developed. At the start of this phase, besides needs-inquiry workshops, individual interviews on background characteristics and environmental features were conducted, as well as some tests to assess the cognitive abilities and disabilities, together with ways of coping and autonomy of the participants. This information was used to specify the functional requirements of the CDN (see also Chapter 7). In total 17 persons suffering from mild dementia of the Alzheimer type participated in the workshops and interviews. After a period of technological development a field test was carried out with the first version of the CDN. During this field test the CDNv-1 was presented to 16 people with mild dementia and their carers in their own home. We will describe how the inventoried disabilities of the people with dementia and their background and environmental features impacted on the functional requirements of the CDN and the opinions of persons with dementia and carers on the user friendliness and usefulness of the developed device.

8.2   The People with Mild Dementia that Participated in the First Phase of the COGKNOW Project

8.2.1   Group Characteristics

In Amsterdam (NL), Belfast (UK) and Luleå (SWE) workshops and interviews were held with persons with dementia and their carers to inventory their needs and to discuss possible and preferred ICT solutions with them. The participants were recruited from memory clinics and/or meeting centres or day care centres for people with dementia and their carers. All persons with dementia in this project suffered from mild dementia of the Alzheimer type with a MMSE score (Mini Mental State Examination, Folstein et al. 1975) between 14 and 25 and/or a Global Deterioration Scale score (Reisberg et al. 1982) of 3, 4 or 5. This involves moderate cognitive decline (late confusional state) and moderately severe cognitive decline (early dementia stage).

At the time of the workshops and interviews all persons with dementia lived in the community and had an informal carer who was also willing to participate in the project. In Table 8.1 some characteristics of the people who participated in the workshops and interviews are presented.

Table 8.1   Characteristics of participants in the needs-inquiry workshops and interviews in the first year of the COGKNOW project

	Amsterdam (n = 6)	Belfast (n = 6)	Luleå (n = 5)	Total (n = 17)
Persons with dementia				
Mean age (years)	64.0 (range 56–78)	72.7 (range 65–86)	67.8 (range 60–77)	68.19 (range 56–86)
Gender	3 female 3 male	5 female 1 male	3 female 2 male	11 female 6 male
Civil status	5 married 1 divorced	3 married 2 widowed 1 single	5 married	13 married 1 divorced 2 widowed 1 single
Carers				
Mean age (years)	58.5 (range 49–78)	53.0 (range 40–72)	61.4 (range 23–78)	57.41 (range 23–78)
Gender	4 female 2 male	3 female 3 male	2 female 3 male	9 female 8 male
Relation to patient	5 spouses 1 daughter	3 spouses 2 children 1 cousin	4 spouses 1 son	12 spouses 1 daughter 2 children 1 cousin 1 son

8.2.2 Methods to Assess Disabilities and Other Relevant Features

Separate needs-inquiry workshops were conducted for persons with dementia and for informal/formal carers at each test site. If preferred by users, individual needs-inquiry interviews were conducted. During the workshops people were asked about their priority of needs and preferred ICT solutions. Powerpoint presentations were used to structure the discussion on experienced disabilities and needs related to specific activities at different times during the day and on preferred solution areas and possible ICT solutions. To stimulate the discussion further a needs and solutions list of a variety of needs of people with dementia and possible ICT solutions in the four COGKNOW areas was presented, based on recent literature (Dröes et al. 2005).

In Amsterdam, two workshops were organized: one with people with dementia and the other with the carers. The workshops were guided by a workshop leader, a senior researcher (psychologist), while a junior researcher (psychologist) assisted and took notes. One couple could not participate in the workshop and was therefore interviewed at home. In Belfast, the method of individual home-based couple interviews was used, as this was felt to be culturally more acceptable and avoided the need for people to discuss their circumstances and problems in an open workshop setting. The interviews therefore took the form of domiciliary visits by two research nurses. Due to the nature of some of the information to be collected, both patient and carer were interviewed individually as well as together. In Luleå most persons with dementia also preferred being individually interviewed. Some people with dementia and carers participated in a small group interview. All interviews were conducted by a senior researcher (social informatics scientist).

After the needs-inquiry workshops individual interviews were conducted at the home of the person with dementia with both the persons with dementia and their carers. During these interviews background characteristics of the person with dementia and carer and environmental features were inventoried, and some tests and questionnaires were administered to assess the cognitive (dis)abilities, ways of coping, quality of life, (experienced) autonomy of the persons with dementia, social network, use of services and unmet needs. The following standardized tests and questionnaires were used (see also Chapter 12):

- Background characteristics of persons with dementia and carers: Standard questionnaire.
- Cognitive abilities/disabilities: The CAMCOG, cognitive test of the Cambridge Examination for mental disorders of the elderly (Roth et al. 1986).
- Deterioration in daily activities: Interview for Deterioration in Daily living activities in Dementia (IDDD) (Teunisse and Derix 1991).
- Ways of coping: Dementia Coping Scale (Reinersmann et al. 2006) and the Jalowiec Coping Scale (Jalowiec 1987, 1991; Dröes 1996; Dröes et al. 2006).
- Quality of life: Quality of life in Alzheimer's disease (QOL-AD; patient and family version) (Logsdon et al. 1999).
- Experienced autonomy: Standardized interview with person with dementia specifically composed for the COGKNOW project (Meiland and Dröes 2006).

- Contextual information: Observation based on checklist and interviews with person with dementia and carer.
- Social network: Practitioners Assessment of Network Type (PANT) questionnaire (Wenger and Tucker 2002).
- Information on received care: List use of services (administered with carer) (Dröes 1996; Schulz 1991).
- Needs and wants potential users: Literature study and Camberwell Assessment of Need for the Elderly (CANE). (Reynolds et al. 2000; translated into Dutch by Dröes et al. 2004).

8.2.3 Disabilities of Participants

The workshops and interviews resulted in an overview of disabilities and needs that the persons with dementia experienced and that had to be taken into account during the development of the CDN (see Hettinga et al. 2007). Unfortunately, not all of the participants were able to answer every question. The total numbers therefore differ between items (this is noted where relevant).

It must be stressed that the findings presented here were based on a small sample of people with mild dementia. No quantitative conclusions can therefore be drawn from them. The needs and disabilities mentioned, as well as the proposed ways to support them, should be considered as examples of needs and disabilities that can occur in people with mild dementia and examples of possible solutions.

In this cohort more than half of the persons with dementia had *problems with memory and orientation in time* and as a consequence needed to be reminded of their appointments. Reminders were therefore expected to be very useful in combination with a fixed place where people could see the time, day and date. Some persons with dementia (in this cohort, 5 out of 16) had *difficulties with verbal instructions*. Their comprehension appeared relatively poor. Simple written instructions on the other hand were understood by all of the persons with dementia in this cohort. Therefore, ICT solutions like the CDN could not depend too heavily on verbal or written instruction and had to make the device as intuitive to use as possible. If instructions were to be used this had to be very simple. In this cohort, 6 out of 16 persons with dementia had problems with *recognizing pictures* and/or *expressing themselves verbally*. With respect to the device to be developed it was therefore clear that simple pictures had to be employed to help people understand the different functions of the buttons of the CDN. Furthermore, a combination of verbal or written instructions together with pictures might be even more helpful. As common in patients with dementia, almost half of the persons with dementia (7 out of 16) experienced (some) *problems with handling objects* (apraxia). This meant that the CDN device should not require complex operation, if to be used independently by persons with dementia. The ICT device needed to be as straightforward as possible to operate. Most persons with dementia were mobile in their close neighbourhood, but 12 out of 17 persons with dementia in this study did have problems in *finding their way in their outside surroundings*. As a consequence, the ICT device preferably had to provide some outdoor navigation support. A mobile CDN device with GPS could therefore be helpful in finding the way home.

Since 6 out of 17 persons with dementia reported to have *difficulties with performing everyday activities*, it would be helpful if the device were to offer instrumental support with everyday activities, for instance, by reminding the person with dementia to carry out certain activities, or with some instruction advice, e.g. on how to use a microwave.

8.2.4 Relevant Background Characteristics and Environmental Features

Apart from the disabilities that people with dementia experience, the usability of ICT devices may also be influenced by personal and environmental features concerning, e.g. living alone or with a carer, physical health and housing situation. We will here describe some of these features.

In the COGKNOW cohort, three persons with dementia *lived alone without a carer*. This meant that they could not rely on support from their carer in operating the developed technological device. To increase the chance of independent usage, any device to support them therefore had to be easy accessible and easy to learn how to operate.

Dementia is primarily a disease of the aged and is therefore accompanied frequently by *other diseases and common complaints of old age*. Participants in the COGKNOW project suffered from varying diseases, such as diabetes, hypertension, stomach ulcer and Parkinson's disease, besides the dementia. It must therefore be stressed that any ICT solution should make things easier, not harder for them, in the context of co-existing morbidities. For example, it is obvious that for people who are suffering from arthritis a lightweight mobile device would be much more user friendly than a heavy weight one.

The participating persons with dementia lived in various *types of housing* and some had different levels in their house. As a consequence, the device to be developed preferably had to be usable in different rooms, e.g. by application of a stationary part in the main (e.g. living) room and a mobile device in other rooms. In cases of multilevel housing, some safety support via sensorized lightning of the corridor and/or staircase at night also seemed desirable. Some (two) persons with dementia suggested the use of night lights that automatically switch on when leaving the bed would also help them to feel safer.

It is not unusual that older persons with dementia use certain *aids* to help them to get around. In the COGKNOW cohort one participant used a cane on which he was quite dependent. It would therefore be helpful if the cane could be marked by a sensor which the ICT device could locate in case the person with dementia could not find it. This principle would of course also be helpful to locate other objects, such as purse, wallet and keys.

All persons with dementia in this cohort had several household equipments (like a microwave, a cooker, an oven, a dishwasher and a washing machine), but most of them had difficulties using them because of *problems with instrumental daily activities*. A device that could offer a stepwise simple automatic explanation on how to use these household appliances was perceived as being potentially helpful.

Most persons with dementia also possessed *other technological appliances,* such as a radio, TV, CD player and mobile phone, but most of them appeared to have problems with operating them and therefore their use was limited. From the 12 persons with dementia that had a mobile phone, only 4 of them could use it and they often forgot to take it with them when going outdoors. Any device to support making phone calls therefore preferably had to use only very simple technology with limited buttons or pictures for dialling. A "find mobile" service to locate the mobile in the house and a reminder to take the mobile when going outdoors also seemed necessary.

Even though 13 persons with dementia of this cohort had access to a *computer,* only 3 of them made use of it since it was too complicated for them. This again stresses the fact that developed technology for this target group has to be made as simple as possible. Finally, in this group only one person with dementia had a PDA (personal data assistant), but he did not use it. Based on these findings one must conclude that when developing a PDA for persons with dementia, the simplicity of the functionality will determine the extent of engagement and use of the device.

Persons with dementia and carers explicitly expressed *their need for company and social contact* with family or friends: 4 persons with dementia and 9 carers mentioned they wanted to have more contact with friends; 13 carers indicated that they had sufficient contacts, but they wanted to maintain these also in the future. An ICT solution, that could help persons with dementia engage in social contact in a simple manner, was therefore expected to be very helpful.

Furthermore, half of the persons with dementia and carers mentioned that they would like the person with dementia to be supported in doing things for fun or recreation. It would therefore be worthwhile to develop an ICT solution that could help them with this, for instance, a simple controllable music player that would enable persons with dementia to listen to their favourite music.

8.3 Functional Requirements Compensating for Disabilities and Personal and Environmental Factors

Based on the inventoried disabilities, needs and wishes of the persons with dementia and the described personal and environmental features, it was concluded that if the device to be developed had to be independently used by persons with dementia, it had to be easy accessible, easy to understand and simple to operate. It was decided to integrate the different functionalities in one system composed of a stationary and a mobile component so that people could use the device and its functions in all rooms of the house. Intuitive usage, with only simple instructions and clear pictures, seemed preferable and the device had to be based on very basic technology. The possible physical complaints of persons with dementia had to be taken into account during the design of the device. Besides these general functional requirements, more detailed requirements for the domains of memory support, social support, activity support and safety support were specified as well (see below).

8.3.1 Supporting Memory

Forgetting appointments affected the lives of all participants. An ICT device that helps in reminding appointments and planning activities was therefore expected to be very useful by the persons with dementia and their carers. To this end, a *simple electronic agenda or calendar* was proposed in which reminders could be remotely configured (e.g. by the carer). Since persons with dementia can experience difficulty in understanding instructions, all textual reminders of appointments and activities had to be formulated as simple as possible (e.g. "it's time for lunch") and preferably be accompanied by a simple picture.

As problems with forgetting appointments can be partly caused by time orientation problems, it was proposed to include a clearly visible *clock and day indicator* in the CDN. As persons with dementia often tend to lose objects, or are afraid of losing them, it was proposed to include some kind of *item locator* in the CDN as well.

8.3.2 Supporting Social Contact

To stay in contact, with beloved ones and the social network, is a generally expressed need and persons with dementia are no exception. However, because of memory and time orientation problems, persons with dementia tend to forget to call family and friends or forget that they had an appointment. Because of problems in handling the equipments (apraxia), they can also have difficulty performing complex instrumental activities like phone calls. One of the possible and presently available ways to support persons with dementia in maintaining social contact is to provide them with a simple *picture-dialling phone* that allows them to make a phone call simply by touching a clear picture of the person they wish to call. It was therefore suggested to integrate a picture telephone in the CDN to support the persons with dementia in maintaining social contact. To help them to remember their appointments with family and friends, it was proposed to offer *reminders for appointments* in both (simple) textual and sound modalities (sound alert).

8.3.3 Supporting Activities in Daily Life

There were several problems stated during the workshops and interviews that expressed the difficulty persons with dementia have with daily activities. For example, persons with dementia frequently forgot that they had planned to undertake a particular activity. The suggested *electronic agenda* was regarded as potentially very helpful for this problem. For instance, a reminder of an appointment to attend a meeting at the community centre could pop up half an hour before the person with dementia had to leave. Reminders to get some bread at the bakery could also be helpful, as well as reminders to stimulate and manage hobbies that are still of interest to the person with dementia. Again simple written reminders accompanied by pictures were stressed.

Another problem mentioned was that when persons with dementia wanted to undertake an activity, they experienced problems reflecting difficulty in planning and sequencing the activity. This occurred especially when trying to use electronic equipment. It was therefore suggested to let the CDN offer *instrumental activity support* by simple stepwise instruction on video on how to execute complex activities, for example, preparing food in a microwave or preparing a cup of coffee.

Because of the problems some persons with dementia had with operating recreational appliances, e.g. turning on the radio or CD player, it was suggested that the CDN would offer a simple *media player function* that allowed people to listen to their preferred music or listen to the radio.

Finally, it was expected that people would go outside more often when they were supported by means of a *GPS-based navigation programme* on the mobile component of the CDN, a so-called Take Me Home service.

8.3.4 Supporting Feelings of Safety

Some persons with dementia declared that they regularly experienced feelings of insecurity. In those cases it would be helpful if the CDN could offer a way to directly contact someone that could offer assistance, e.g. the primary carer. Therefore, it was suggested to include a help button on the CDN, both on the stationary and on the mobile component. This would allow people to ask for help when they experience problems and to feel more secure even while being outdoors.

Another way to enhance feelings of safety is to employ sensor-based warnings. For example, by means of a sensor at the front door, or the fridge door, a warning can be given to help people remember that they have to close the door if left open. It was suggested to include this functionality in the CDN as a further measure to enhance safety.

To enhance feelings of safety during the night a sensorised night lamp was proposed that would automatically switch on when people went out of bed.

8.4 Opinions on User Friendliness and Usefulness of the CDNv-1

After specifying the preferred functional requirements, checking on the technical feasibility with the technological developers, and prioritizing functionalities to be developed in the first and following project years, eventually eight functionalities in four support domains were selected as the focus for the first field test with users (see Table 8.2).

Table 8.2 Functionalities for COGKNOW Day Navigator in field test #1

1. Reminding functionality
   a. locator for the mobile device
   b. textual reminders for food intake, brush teeth, make phone calls, appointments, charge mobile
   c. day and time indication
2. Picture-dialling functionality
3. Functionality for activity support
   a. turn on/off radio via touch screen
   b. media playback
4. Safety support functionality
   a. a warning is given when the door is left open/unlocked
   b. easy emergency contact

Several weeks before the field test a pretest interview was arranged with the person with dementia and carer (i) to check if participants still fulfilled the inclusion criteria, (ii) to confirm informed consent, (iii) to make appointments on practical procedures during the field test and (iv) to collect information necessary to configure the reminders in the agenda, the pictures in the address book and the preferred music in the media playback player.

In total 16 persons with dementia and carers participated in the field tests in Amsterdam, Belfast and Luleå. Two of the 17 persons with dementia that participated in the workshops dropped out in the field tests (one person in Amsterdam because of cognitive deterioration meaning he no longer fulfilled the inclusion criterion of "mild" dementia anymore (MMSE <14) and the other person in Belfast withdrew consent). In Luleå one new person with dementia was recruited for the field test.

The field tests were carried out in 1 day, except for two persons with dementia in Luleå who used the CDN for a period of 6 days. After installation of the device in the home of the person with dementia, the different functionalities on the stationary and mobile component of the CDN were demonstrated, and persons with dementia were trained in using the device with the help of a small user manual. After that persons with dementia were asked to conduct several prescribed tasks with regard to each functionality and to give their opinion on the user friendliness and usefulness of each of the functions. To standardize the procedure for the three test sites, semi-structured interviews and an observation scheme were used. After finishing the test with the person with dementia, the carer was interviewed as well on the perceived user friendliness and usefulness of the device for the person with dementia. During the test the researchers also completed a bottle-neck list.

The overall opinion of the persons with dementia and carers on the CDN was that the device was user friendly and easy to operate and that its functionalities were useful.

General design and layout: There were some people who made comments on the external design of the stationary device. They suggested it could be adapted to blend in better with the furniture in their living room. Several persons with dementia felt that not all of the screen icons were clear (e.g. the help button and find mobile icon) and they therefore suggested to the use of more easily recognizable and clearer icons to represent specific functionalities. Some carers proposed a wall-mounted CDN device as persons with dementia often tend to move things around and they thought the persons with dementia would become more easily accustomed to a fixed device.

Reminding functionality: The audibility of the reminding system was judged as sufficient. Some of the users commented that it would be helpful if the text reminders were accompanied by flashing screens and/or a sound signal to attract the attention of the person with dementia.

The user friendliness of the text reminders seemed to be appropriate on the home screen, but readability decreased on the mobile device. It was believed that the usefulness of the reminders could be enhanced by personalizing them with respect to content, text and clear pictures and by an attempt to attune them to the individual needs of persons with dementia.

Carers liked the idea of being able to easily configure the reminders themselves in the electronic agenda.

Picture-dialling functionality: The picture-dialling facility was evaluated as user friendly by most of the persons with dementia and carers. They found it easy to operate and easy to learn how to use it. The usefulness of this service was ranked high. According to the users, the user friendliness would increase if individual adaptations of the address book could be made (e.g. increasing or decreasing the number of addresses). There were some persons with dementia who had difficulty recognizing the small-size pictures on the mobile device. Suggestions were also made to diminish the different steps necessary for dialling. There appeared to be some confusion about the aim of the help button as people used it as an easy way to start a general phone call with the informal carer. This could be prevented by using another icon for the help button, for example, a life safer ring to emphasize that the button was meant to be used in case of urgency. Some persons with dementia suggested to integrate the telephone horn at the (right or left) side of the stationary screen. The positive evaluation of the picture-dialling function confirmed that people with mild dementia can still learn to use simple equipment.

Functionality for activity support: The media control (radio on/off) and media playback (preselected music) functions were rated user friendly by both persons with dementia and carers. However, the quality of the radio reception was sometimes poor. To improve the usefulness of the functionality, it was suggested that easy configuration of personally selected music and selection of different radio stations become a possible option. Some other additional functionality was suggested as well, such as TV control.

Safety support functionality: Only a partial test of safety functionality was possible during the field tests because of technical problems. In Luleå, a door sensor was tested and judged by the persons with dementia as possibly useful in the future, but not at that moment. It was suggested to install a camera that was linked to the stationary screen at the entrance door, allowing for assistance in the identification of visitors.

As an added functionality, an automatic switch-off device for the cooker was suggested. Both persons with dementia and carers stated that this would enhance their feelings of safety and feelings of autonomy of the person with dementia.

8.5 Conclusions

In this chapter we described how disabilities and other relevant features can be taken into account when developing assistive technological devices for people with dementia. We used the COGKNOW project as a case example. Within the COGKNOW project assistive technology is being developed to support people with mild dementia in the areas of memory, social contact, activity and safety. To this end the so-called COGKNOW Day Navigator (CDN) is in the process of development. To make a user friendly and useful device a user-driven design is being applied in which the technological development is based on the needs, wishes and cognitive disabilities and abilities of the target group. To inventory these literature studies, need-inquiry workshops and individual interviews were conducted with people with mild dementia and their carers in Amsterdam, Belfast and Luleå, before the actual technological development of the device took place. To our knowledge, this strategy reflects a rather unique process since most ICT-based services for people with dementia are developed with little input from the target users themselves; many are tested or evaluated via single case studies or small sample sizes of people with dementia (Lauriks et al. 2007). Within COGKNOW we use a relatively large and varied European sample size which provides a lot of information on the possible variations in disabilities, circumstances and needs of persons with dementia that are relevant for the development and acceptance of assistive technology.

The main dementia-related disabilities in the first year COGKNOW cohort that proved relevant for the development of the CDN were memory and orientation problems, poor understanding of verbal instruction and difficulty with instrumental daily activities and as a consequence limited in their operation of technical appliances. Further more, participants had difficulty in recognising the meaning of pictures (e.g. used to indicate functionalities on the touch screen). Relevant personal and environmental features were living alone or with a carer, the need for company and social contact, the need for support in doing things for fun or recreation, using aids like a cane, possessing technological appliances that could not be easily used anymore, living in a house with multiple rooms and levels and feeling insecure when alone.

To compensate for the mentioned disabilities, assistive technology was developed that first reminds people of appointments and activities through the use of simple textual reminders combined with clear icons and a sound alert and second assists temporal orientation via a day and time indicator. To support persons with dementia that had difficulty with instrumental daily activities in maintaining social contact and doing things for fun or recreation, a picture-dialling function, an easy to operate media playback function and a radio on/off control function were included in the device.

Taken into account the relevant personal and environmental features, the aim was to develop a device that is easy to understand and independent to operate by people with mild dementia, can be used mainly intuitively, with only simple instruction and is easily accessible at different places indoors and outdoors by means of a stationary and a mobile component. To help enhance feelings of security, sensor-based safety warnings were introduced and a help button was included to be used in case of urgent need of assistance.

The inventoried disabilities and personal and environmental features greatly helped to specify the functional requirements of a user friendly and useful device for this target group. This was confirmed in the user field tests. Most persons with dementia and carers proved satisfied with the CDNv-1 and its functionalities and found it mostly easy to understand and operate and useful. There were also some suggestions for improvement, such as personalization of reminders with text and clear pictures, layout, preselected music, decreasing the steps in the picture-dialling function and increasing the size of pictures on the mobile phone. The latter suggestion was also made in a pilot study into the user friendliness and effect of mobile coaching in people with dementia (Kort 2005). It became evident that the variety of interests, disabilities and environmental factors make tuning of the device to the needs of individual persons with dementia necessary. A challenge in the second iteration of the project would therefore be to further develop the personalization possibility of the CDN and its functions.

While the CDN is able to help people with mild dementia in certain domains like reminding and remembering, social contact, daily activity and feelings of safety, it also has limitations. For example, persons with dementia and their carers stated that they needed more safety measures during cooking, such as an automatic switch-off for the gas. Unfortunately this is very hard to accomplish within the framework of the COGKNOW project, since stoves and cookers in the different European countries where the field tests are executed are not universally compatible. Another often mentioned demand was to use reminders for medicine intake. We decided not to investigate this option yet, because of safety reasons (lack of control on the actual medicine intake). When the COGKNOW Day Navigator is completely operational new modules could possibly be added to further increase the usefulness in the different need areas.

Nevertheless, since the usefulness and user friendliness were judged positively by persons with dementia and carers, we expect the CDN to be widely applicable in supporting people with mild dementia to navigate through their day, especially when it is improved based on the comments made by persons with dementia and carers. One of the preconditions of the effective and safe use of the CDN by persons with dementia would be a technically stable and reliable device. Only a dependable, high-quality product that persons with dementia can rely on will help to motivate them to actually use it in their daily life.

The first iteration of the COGKNOW project showed that persons with dementia and their carers differ in their respective views on needs and wants of the person with dementia as well as the preferred assistive technology solutions that might provide useful assistance. Therefore it is advisable to let both persons with dementia and carers participate in the development process to inventory opinions from both their perspectives (see also Lauriks et al. 2007). This study showed that people with mild dementia are very well able to give their opinion on the (unmet) needs they experience in daily life and on possible ICT support and to participate in the development and evaluation of assistive technology.

References

ASTRID. (2000) ASTRID: A Guide to Using Technology Within Dementia Care. Hawker publications, London.

Dröes, R.M. (1996) Amsterdamse Ontmoetingscentra; een nieuwe vorm van ondersteuning voor mensen met dementie en hun verzorgers. [Amsterdam Meeting Centers; a New Method of Support for People with Dementia and Their Carers]. Thesis Publishers, Amsterdam.

Dröes, R.M., Meiland, F.J.M., Doruff, S., Varodi, I., Akkermans, H., Baida, Z., Faber, E., Haaker, T., Moelaert, F., Kartseva, V., Tan, Y.H. (2005) A dynamic interactive social chart in dementia care: Attuning demand and supply in the care for persons with dementia and their carers. Studies in Health Technology and Informatics, 114:210–220.

Dröes, R.M., Meiland, F.J.M., van Tilburg, W. (March 2006) Effect of the Meeting Centres Support Program of informal carers of people with dementia: Results form a multi-centre study. Aging Mental Health, 10(2):112–124.

Dröes, R.M., van Hout, H.P.J., van de Ploeg, E.S. (2004) Camberwell Assessment of Need for the Elderly (CANE). Revised version IV. Dutch translation. VU University medical center, Amsterdam.

Folstein, M.F., Folstein, S.E., McHugh, P.R. (1975) "Mini-mental state". A practical method for grading the cognitive state of patients for the clinician. Journal of Psychiatric Research, 12: 189–198.

Hettinga, M., Andersson, A.L., Dröes, R.M., Meiland, F.J., Armstrong, E., Bergvall-Kåreborn, B., Bresciani, M., Craig, D., Sävenstedt, S., Davies, R., van Eijk, R., Johnston, H., Nugent, C., Bengtsson, J.E. (April 2007) Functional Requirements Specification Field Test 1 (COGKNOW D1.4.1.), M. Hettinga (ed.). Telematica Insituut, Enschede.

Jalowiec, A. (1987) Jalowiec Coping Scale (revised version of 1977). Loyola University, Chicago.

Jalowiec, A. (1991) Psychometric Results on the 1987 Jalowiec Coping Scale. School of Nursing, Loyola University, Chicago.

Kort, S. (2005) Mobile Coaching. A pilot study into the user friendliness and effects of Mobile Coaching on the wellbeing of people with dementia and their informal caregivers. MSc thesis, Faculty of Psychology, Vrije Universiteit, Amsterdam.

Lauriks, S., Reinersmann, A., van der Roest, H.G., Meiland, F.J.M., Davies, R.J., Moelaert, F., Mulvenna, M.D., Nugent, C.D., Dröes, R.M. (2007) Review of ICT-based services for identified unmet needs in people with dementia. Ageing Research Reviews, 6:223–246.

Logsdon, R.G., Gibbons, L.E., McCurry, S.M., Teri, L. (1999) Quality of life in Alzheimer's disease: Patient and caregiver reports. Journal of Mental Health and Aging, 5(1): 21–32.

Meiland, F.J.M., Dröes, R.M. (2006) Experienced Autonomy. VU University Medical Center, Department of Psychiatry, EMGO Institute, Amsterdam.

Orpwood, R., Gibbs, C., Adlam, T., Faulkner, R. (2005) The design of smart homes for people with dementia – User interface aspects. In: S. Keates, P. Clarkson, P. Langdon, P. Robinson (eds.) Design for a More Inclusive World. Special issue of Universal Access in the Information Society, 4:156–164.

Reinersmann, A., Meiland, F.J.M., Dröes, R.M. (2006) Dementia Coping Scale. Internal Publication, VU University Medical Center, Amsterdam.

Reisberg, B., Ferris, S., De Leon, M.J., Crook, T. (1982) The Global Deterioration Scale for assessment of primary degenerative dementia. American Journal of Psychiatry, 139(9):1136–1139.

Reynolds, T., Thornicroft, G., Abas, M. et al. (2000) Camberwell Assessment of Need for the Elderly (CANE): Development, validity and reliability. British Journal of Psychiatry, 176: 444–452.

Roth, M., Tym, E., Mountjoy, C.Q., Huppert, F.A., Hendrie, H., Verma, S., Goddard, R. (1986) CAMDEX A standardised instrument for the diagnosis of mental disorder in the elderly with special reference to the early detection of dementia. British Journal of Psychiatry, 149:698–709.

Schultz, C. (1991) Dementie onderzoek; een verkennende studie naar de verzorgers van dementerende bejaarden in Amsterdam. Internal Publication, Psychiatric Center Amsterdam/Valeriuskliniek, Amsterdam.

Sixsmith, A.J., Gibson, G., Orpwood, R.D., Torrington, J.M. (2007) Developing a technology 'wish-list' to enhance the quality of life of people with dementia. Gerontechnology, 6:2–19.

Teunisse, S., Derix, M.M. (1991) Meten van het dagelijks functioneren van thuiswonende dementiepatiënten: Ontwikkeling van een vragenlijst. Gerontology and Geriatrics, 22:53–59.

Wenger, G.C., Tucker, I. (January 2002) Using network variation in practice: Identification of support network type. Health and Social Care in the Community, 10(1):28–35.

Part III
Pervasive Healthcare Technology

Chapter 9
The Role of Context-Aware Computing in Support of People with Dementia

Matthias Baumgarten and Maurice D. Mulvenna

Abstract There is a strong motivation, in particular in the domain of healthcare, for new perspectives on context-driven research and computing in order to provide next-generation services to people that are tailored to individual needs rather than generalised assumptions that could potentially endanger human life. For that, context awareness is a key requirement in order to reach a better understanding of human-centric computing systems and environments, and subsequently, the deployment of dedicated services that are specifically adapted to the context to which they are applied. Such context-driven services would be able to provide the means of delivering situation-aware and person-centric services that ultimately may even anticipate future behaviour and problems of the user itself and the context in which the user finds themselves. However, the perpetual provision of contextual data in pervasive environments is far from being easy and includes major challenges that vary between environments. The reason for this is not only the sensor diversity within the environments themselves but also the contextual scope to be analysed and the amount of data to be collected and correlated to actually reach a minimum degree of contextual understanding. For that reason, in this chapter, contextual environments have been categorised as well as their interaction into different groups that reflect individual contextual levels of interest of which contextual understanding is required and consequently to which services can be applied.

9.1 Introduction

On a worldwide context the human population continues to grow rapidly with an increasing percentage represented by the elderly. Considering that the elderly have a higher likelihood of requiring care for various conditions and illnesses, society

M. Baumgarten (✉)
TRAIL Living Lab, School of Computing and Mathematics, Faculty of Computing and Engineering, University of Ulster, Newtownabbey, Northern Ireland
e-mail: m.baumgarten@ulster.ac.uk

M.D. Mulvenna, C.D. Nugent (eds.), *Supporting People with Dementia Using Pervasive Health Technologies*, Advanced Information and Knowledge Processing, DOI 10.1007/978-1-84882-551-2_9, © Springer-Verlag London Limited 2010

is faced with the increasing problem of providing good and cost-effective health-care on an ever-growing scale. In the UK alone it is estimated that well over a million people will suffer from dementia by 2025 with associated financial cost of over 17 billion pounds (Alzheimers Organisation 2009). Two-third of people with dementia still live in the community and the vast majority of all would like to continue to do so. Thus, there is a general shift from institutional to community care which, however, requires substantial restructuring of healthcare infrastructures and their service provisions. In particular, automated supervision and reinforcement mechanisms could provide the means to enable people in general but in particular people with dementia to remain within their local environment without the constant presence of a human caretaker. The resulting preventative services could help to maintain social interactions, provide assistance and guidance for daily life activities but most importantly they could provide an automated safety network that enables people to remain independent in their own home environment. Nevertheless, in order to provide such services a workable balance has to be found between peoples' needs and the introduction and utilisation of ubiquitous computing environments and the services they facilitate.

Through the deployment of latest sensor technology the move towards "home automation", smart or intelligent environments can be considered to be one that promotes levels of independence and increases personal autonomy (Helal et al. 2003) by being able to deliver services in a context and situation-aware manner.

Within this chapter the role of context-aware computing can play in supporting independent living is evaluated. The chapter also explores how it can be used to improve the quality of life for various aspects. In particular and within the first part of the chapter, the conceptual aspects of individual context-aware environments will be discussed and the possible types of interactions will be outlined. The second part will discuss the potential for contextual reasoning and context prediction within such environments and will also provide a number of service categories for which a virtually unlimited number of tasks could be devised for and that would support various aspects of daily life activities.

9.2 Context-Aware Computing

The challenge for ubiquitous and pervasive computing is in managing a sophisticated and dynamic perspective on computer-mediated interactions with human beings without intruding unnecessarily into their lives. This is what is described as the notion of calm (Weiser 1991), where computing resources quietly modify themselves to suit the needs of the user. In order to make sense of ubiquitous computing environments, the word context has been used to describe how sensors, processors and actuators can interpret and influence the environment. As recognised in Dey (2001), the term context has been defined differently for different domains and moreover it may also mean different things to different people. The term context-aware computing has arisen from a well-established body of ubiquitous computing research concerned with location (Schilit et al. 1994). It was defined in the context of the systems in which the user employs many different mobile, embedded and stationary computers in different situations and locations over the course of the day. This has evolved from within several research fields sharing many common views, including ubiquitous computing (Weiser 1991; Dey and Abowd 1999), pervasive computing (Ark and Selker 1999) and ambient intelligence (Aarts and Collier 2003) where the term context refers to any information that can be used to characterise the situation of a person or a computational entity. Although, weak in a sense that it lacks a formal definition and instead includes practically all information, meaningful or not, in this chapter the latter definition is supported given the context of ambient intelligence. The reason for that is simply based on the fact that a given context can in fact be influenced by "any information". Thus, it is in fact the application that usually defines the scope of the context desired and not the environment. That is of course in dependence to the information that are available to the application. Note that depending on issues related to security, privacy, etc. some information available in the environment may be hidden from the application and as such cannot be used by it.

Research in human–computer interaction such as Dourish (2004) proposes a perspective on context-aware computing where the context is perceived much as in social sciences that study the practices of individuals in their normal environment. Here, the problem of context is examined from a high level, philosophical point of view, highlighting an approach that views context as an interactional problem rather than a representational one. Another form is that of dynamic contexts (Sterritt et al. 2005) where it is the activity that generates and sustains the context. So, context arises from the activity and is actively produced and maintained in the course of the activity. This provides a framework for a method to determine context from activity via behaviour (and measures of behaviour) and is in line with the research vision of Suchmann (1987). Indeed, the perspective of context arising from interactions is very close to the vision of research from those researching socially aware computing and communication, where social computing proposes ubiquitous computing environments and resources that understand social signalling and social context (Pentland 2005).

In order to manage context events, a framework is needed that supports the management of extensible context and context histories and makes it possible to utilise context in context-aware environments. However, it seems that there is no consensus for context or context history utilisation (capturing, representing, modelling and using context) over time. The development of research into context histories (Helander 2005; Wilson et al. 2005; Schneider et al. 2005) provides an important framework for higher level representation of labelled contexts and is a foundation for emerging research in such areas as the continuous archival and retrieval of personal experiences (e.g. Aizawa et al. 2004) as famously described in Bush (1945). Some practical problems include the fact that acquired information can be strongly heterogeneous and often incorrect, inconsistent or incomplete and, worse of all, not at all or insufficiently correlated with each other. A second issue is that context is used in systems in various ways which makes it difficult to understand if it is stored "out of context". A substantial number of different approaches have been proposed to model such contextual information. The most sophisticated propose a form of layered context structure framework, with a context provider layer for the incorporation of raw sensor and actuator data and a context service layer for context provision in context-aware environments (Huebscher and McCann 2005). This would allow for facilitating some form of computational model of context processing as in Balkenius and Moren (2000) and Strang and Linnhoff-Popien (2004) that orchestrates context stimuli and components into a single and coherent representation or places the interaction into a practical framework (DiDuca and Van-Helvert 2005). There is also a requirement to gauge the quality of our contextual information and histories objectively as it is gathered, as from the Quality of Context (QoC) mechanism of Buchholz and Kupper (2003), in which any contextual information comes associated with parameters including precision of information, correctness probability, trustworthiness, resolution and recency. Simply said, contextual information cannot be reduced to a trivial set of data to be accessed by components, but requires some higher form of organisation that correlates individual data entities with each other and more importantly with the application itself.

Overall, there is a very clear research roadmap for context-aware computing, driven in many ways by researchers who care a great deal about people and the interaction of people in independent living environments. Providing a true context stack is a significant research challenge and clearly the incorporation of a context reasoning and prediction layer into such a stack could both provide intelligent support and also facilitate strong communication capabilities via social inter-networks of family, friends, peers and others.

9.3 Context Environments

The term smart environment is usually used to refer to sensor-rich infrastructures that allow for the gathering of raw contextual data. The technology deployed within such environments varies from simple sensors over localised environments in order to detect, e.g. a door opening and closing to more elaborate sensor systems that reflect openly accessible smart infrastructures as necessary to achieve full contextual-awareness at various levels of granularity. The information therein may be sampled and monitored locally or remotely providing a framework where decisions can be made in instances of concern where, for instance, a person may require some form of intervention to, e.g. prevent a given situation worsening. In these environments, the technological sensing capability already allows not only to monitor the movements of a person but also their interaction with devices or other stakeholders within the environment. For example, turning the cooker on or off, turning a tap on or off or adjusting the temperature within the home. Such data, if correlated correctly, can then be sequenced into chains of events that can be used to, e.g. advise next actions to be done in order to perform certain tasks. For instance, fill the kettle with water before switching it on. Alternatively, if compared to another event pattern, they can be used to detect unwanted or even dangerous situation before they actually happen. For instance, switching on the oven before going to bed is potentially dangerous and most certainly unwanted. Here an alarm could be raised or the cooker could be switched off automatically via an associated actuator.

Naturally, if desired information cannot be sensed, correlated or reasoned for then they are by default not available for subsequent tasks. Similarly, if a system lacks in understanding of the available information then their usefulness is questionable as the quality cannot be determined. Finally, no single service can address all of the requirements and complexities required in a given domain. Thus, the awareness and utilisation of other services that are available in the same or other environments are important for the success of individual services. Therefore the three core aspects for the successful deployment of contextual services in smart infrastructures can be summarised as (a) the sensing capabilities of the system, (b) the understanding thereof and (c) the services available on the system.

Considering the above and the distributed nature of the underlying sensor-based architecture smart environments may be categorised as follows:

- *Known Macro-environments*: Such environments are limited in a sense that they have clearly defined boundaries with respect to their spatial dimensions and sensorial capabilities. They are known in a way that they are purpose built and as such the type of information and their relation to each other is known. Services deployed in such an environment may take direct advantage of the knowledge that is incorporated in the infrastructure and the standardised interfaces thereof. Probably the most relevant example for such an environment is that of a smart home.
- *Unknown Macro-environments*: Also limited in the same sense as above but may be unknown to the application, service or user that are interacting with the environment. A good example for such an environment would be public smart buildings, e.g. hospitals, schools and parks. Such environments are by default unknown to a potential user and also differ with respect to the sensor and service infrastructure. However, resources deployed would be clearly defined so that the environment could be used exploratory. Here an additional layer would be required that is capable of bridging the gap between the environment and the service that are trying to utilise it.
- *Unknown Openenvironments*: Are defined to have no spatial or sensor (or at least very open) boundaries but are equipped with smart devices that can be accessed by potential users and applications and on which other users can deploy their own services, e.g. the physical layout of a large city may represent such an environment, where spatial boundaries are practically not present and where a multitude of different sensors and services may be available from unknown and as such uncertified sources. In such an environment the mapping between the infrastructure and the services would be very difficult, if not impossible, if no degree of standardisation or contextual description exists.
- *Specialised Micro-environments*: In some cases, small scale and highly specialised environments may also be considered as contextual environments. For

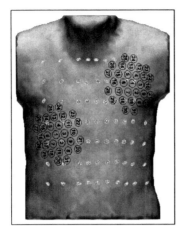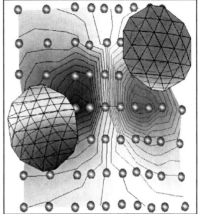

Fig. 9.1 Localised diagnostic environment (Emerald Insight 2009)

instance, Fig. 9.1 depicts a localised diagnostic environment applied to a person. If conditions require the detailed and perpetual monitoring of micro-aspects within a more globally orientated context environment then it would certainly be beneficial if such specialised micro-environments become part of the overall contextual infrastructure, e.g. within this example, a person's cardiac-related bio-signs are constantly measured and may be analysed locally. If connected to a smart home environment, for instance, a person's exercise activity could be performed and synchronised with their current physical condition as measured through the diagnostic system. This would avoid not only that a person is exercising too much but it could also advise to stop exercising if current heart condition would not warrant this.

9.4 Context-Driven Interaction

Similar to the above environment-based categorisation, services can be categorised based on the stakeholders involved or the type of interaction performed. In relation to the environment-based categorisation, the following three categories can be distinguished:

- *People-to-Environment Interaction*: Considering a localised smart environment as depicted in Fig. 9.2a, which illustrates a home environment. The flexible and dynamic interaction between each individual aspect of such an environment and its inhabitants, and vice versa, offers a wide range for possible pervasive services that could help facilitating daily life activities. Similarly, consider a more global-orientated smart world infrastructure such as depicted in Fig. 9.2b. Such

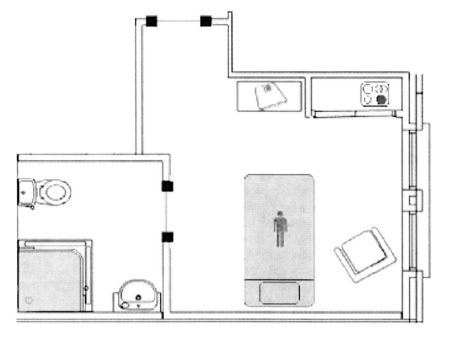

(a) Smart Environment

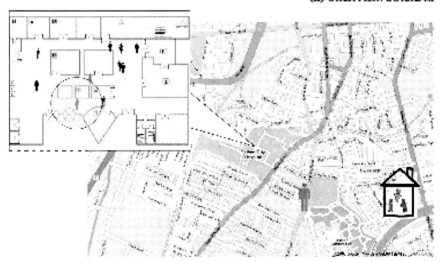

(b) Smart World Infrastructure

Fig. 9.2 People-to-environment interaction

an environment is by far more dynamic, that is, the type and amount of available contextual information are much more diverse and larger, respectively. Furthermore, the types of services to be applied may differ for different locations. For instance, the same type of service in two different towns may produce a different result. As for (a) potential services include the tracking of the person's movement within the house of the use of appliances and for (b) a kind of guideMeTo (Location(x)) service could be used to actually guide a person from a given location to another one, e.g. a hospital for weekly checkups. To ensure the safety of the patient this service would need to interact with localised services such as traffic lights.

- *Environment-to-Environment Interaction*: The interaction between environments themselves or, to be more precise, between the services deployed in them forms another important category of context-driven interaction. Such communication is not only relevant to interlink individual environments but also in instances of mobility, for instance, if a person moves from one environment to another. A "handover" can be initiated that transfers certain services or responsibilities that are relevant to this particular person to the destination environment. Another potentially useful application would be that similar environments could share their "expertise" in order to optimise their own services.

- *People-to-People Interaction*: The interaction between people represents another area where dedicated pervasive services can be applied. In this case specific interactions may be invoked; configured or individual personal interest may be shared to achieve separate goals. The identification of individual interaction entities and the negations of available and needed services represent distinct objectives in this area that would allow for the identification, localisation, spatial guidance and other person-to-person services.

9.5 Towards Context Reasoning and Context Prediction

Context-aware environments will undoubtedly play a vital role in the provision of next-generation person-centric and situation-specific services. However, they also provide the basis for advanced reasoning and prediction capabilities that may lead to intelligent environments that are intrinsically interwoven with services and as such would be able to offer a large degree of intelligent features as required for fully autonomic environments. In particular, such environments would be more flexible with respect to their use; they would be more resilient and failsafe and would in general be able to provide a higher degree of interaction as well as understanding. For instance, if a person detection sensor in a room would fail for any reason, the associated service could reason that "if the door has been opened and the light has been switched on" there is a person in the room. Vice versa, "if the light has been switched off, the door closed and nobody is lying in the bed" then the likelihood that nobody is in this room is high. Obviously, such reasoning is not always failsafe and as such needs to interact with as many information sources as possible to validate individual results from various scenarios. This is of particular interest if individual sensor information contradicts each other. For instance, a sensor embedded in a light switch indicates that the light is switched on. However, a separate light sensor in the same room registers the light to be switched off. Obviously, such a situation would indicate a fault in the senor environment and a reasoning engine could trigger corrective measures. Nevertheless, the question of the light being on or off still remains. In order to answer this question additional sensors would be required that either sense the same concept of the existing sensors, thus introducing a level of redundancy over which a system can reason, or alternatively a separate concept needs to be sensed, which needs, however, to be associated with the problem concerned. For the example discussed the power intake of the room could be measured and correlated with the devices activated in the room in order to determine if the light is actually on or off. In the literature, reasoning tasks can be categorised to be inductive, deductive or abductive. Deductive reasoning is a top-down approach that allows to (in-)validate a theory or condition. For instance, "the light is on" if "light switch = on" and "light sensor = bright". Inductive reasoning on the other hand is a bottom-up approach and seeks a broader generalisation that is based on specific observations. For example, if "light switch = on" and "light sensor = bright" then "the light is on". Finally, adductive reasoning attempts to infer logical explanations based on specific observation. For instance, if "light sensor = bright" then "light switch = on". However, unlike the principles of deduction this statement does not necessarily infer the fact that "the light is on". In abduction the inferred results do not have to be necessarily true in the wider context of the problem that is under scrutiny. Instead they are possible explanations that may be further validated using deduction.

Taking the above into account reasoning can be used to (a) prove hypotheses that lead to generalised rules of behaviour, (b) infer an hypothesis based on observations which in turn can be further validated and (c) explain the dependencies between concepts. Now in order to answer the question of if the light is actually on or off, consider the scenario depicted in Fig. 9.3.

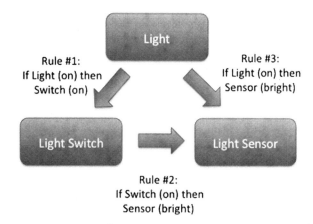

Fig. 9.3 Contextual reasoning

Here the concept under scrutiny is if the light is on or off and the parameters under observation are a light switch and a light sensor. Through common sense two rules have been established stating that if the light is on then the switch is on and that if the switch is on the sensor is sensing bright. Note that Rule #3 is not known beforehand. The goal is to verify that the light is actually on if the switch is set to on. For this consider the following: if the light switch is set to on then it can be, through inductive reasoning and Rule #1, inferred that the light is on. However, at this stage this is only a hypothesis that is not yet proven. Rule #2 states that the sensor is bright if the switch is on which infers, through abductive reasoning, that the sensor is also bright if the light is on. Thus, Rule #3 can be generated. Now, through deductive reasoning it can be argued that the light is indeed on if the switch is set to on *and* if the sensor is sensing bright.

Although very simple, the above scenario illustrates the potential of the various reasoning mechanisms for context-aware environments. In particular the verification of individual contexts in relation to given parameters will depend heavily on such mechanisms.

Another important aspect for context-aware environments is that of context prediction, which in a context-aware environment makes possible proactive devices and device interfaces that go some way towards the provision of a calm environment, as envisaged by Weiser (1991). We define context prediction as the ability to predict the possible future contexts of interaction with people or other contextual environments, as described by Mayerhofer et al. (2003). This means that individual behaviourally based profiles may be accessed and used to understand and manage behaviour traits. However, this is a significant research challenge requiring dynamic, layered, socially orientated and extensible context "stacks" with new research required especially for the definition of a context prediction stack. DiDuca and Van-Helvert (2005) state that "service offerings may be based on such things as rhythms or patterns of behaviour, body language, etc. which suggests that we may have to look beyond mainstream approaches and consider methods from different domains such as ethnographic, observational or pattern recognition approaches." Some research perspectives on possible context architectures provide helpful insights. In particular, Nurmi et al. (2005) reason that context monitoring and reasoning require large amount of resources and to address this issue perhaps distributed and peer-to-peer approaches could be used. We have examined this issue in a related research area (Mulvenna and Zambonelli 2005) and believe that it does show promise, perhaps particularly, in the area of use of semantic overlay technologies as researched in Loeser (2003) and Nurmi et al. (2005) also raises the important issue of prediction sharing, where individuals or their environments may have access to the contexts, context histories and/or context predictions of others. In their research, Petzold et al. focus also on context prediction based on previous behaviour patterns. Their proposed prediction algorithms originate in branch prediction techniques (known from the area of processor architecture), which are transformed to handle context prediction (Petzold and Bagci 2003). Irrespective of the use of predictive mechanism in general it holds that the better the accuracy and the longer the prediction is valid for the more useful it will be for any form of guidance or system adaptation.

9.6 Context-Aware Computing in Support of People with Dementia

With over 5 million people affected by dementia in all of Europe (Alzheimer's Europe 2009) it becomes clear that new and cost-effective ways are needed to provide the best care possible. Providing home support at various levels from an early stage onwards could avoid or at least delay institutionalisation which in turn would increase the quality of life of a patient while simultaneously being more cost-effective. Within an intelligent context-aware environment, a number of different categories of services could be thought of for which virtually an unlimited number of individual services could be deployed that can be used to support a wide range of daily task activities. Figure 9.4 depicts some categories for which various services could be devised that actively reinforce a person's confidence for certain tasks, utilises reminders to guide certain activities, improves and maintains social interaction or helping caretakers and doctors by providing relevant support in relation to the person cared for.

In short, such services do not only have the potential just to increase the confidence and safety a person is experiencing but do have the potential to prolong independent living beyond current threshold. This is particularly relevant for dementia-related care where a person's physical fitness would often allow for an independent lifestyle but cognitive decline may necessitate institutionalisation. By providing relevant guidance and safety layers such that people could live independently for longer would ultimately improve quality of life. In order to realise such services realistically, a generalised framework is required that supports the management of extensible context and context histories and makes it possible to utilise context in ubiquitous environments in a flexible and open manner. However, as

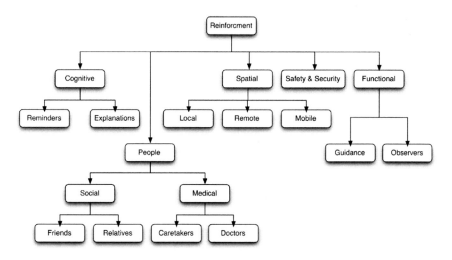

Fig. 9.4 Example of service types supporting daily life activities

stated earlier, there is no general consensus yet for the use of context or context history-related information.

9.7 Conclusion

It has been shown that there is a clear need for intelligent services that are able to support ageing people in general but in particular those people suffering from certain medical conditions such as mild dementia but wish to continue to live independently. The types of services that could be offered in context-aware environments will centre on cognitive and social reinforcement in addition to the functional support for daily activities. Contemporary mobile devices such as personal digital assistants (PDA) or smart phones are already being specifically tailored towards the use by elderly and disabled people so that technology will be actually supporting rather than being an obstacle. The major benefit of such technology is that people can remain in their home environment for longer which will not only be more cost-effective but will also improve the quality of life for the person and the family and friends around them. However, if such services are limited to the home itself then this could lead to the virtual imprisonment of people in their own home. The use of portable technology such as mobile phones can ensure the continuity of services beyond the limits of individual macro-environments. However, to be fully effective, contextual environments have to be made available in a fully pervasive and open fashion at all levels of granularity.

There are valuable lessons from socially orientated research in usability and situated action that has to be incorporated into intelligent context-aware environments for context-aware technology to be successful. This chapter has reviewed and examined layered and extensible context architectures that provide self-managed and self-configuration autonomic capabilities. In addition to the context provider and context service layers, context reasoning and context prediction layers with cross-layer QoC capabilities have been discussed.

References

Alzheimer's Europe. (2009)   www.alzheimer-europe.org, last accessed February 2009.
Alzheimer's Organisation. (2009)   www.alzheimers.org, last accessed February 2009.
Aarts, E., Collier, R. (2003) Ambient intelligence. First European Symposium, EUSAI 2003, Springer, Veldhoven, The Netherlands.
Aizawa, K., Tancharoen, D., Kawasaki, S., Yamasaki, T. (2004) Efficient retrieval of life log based on context and content. The First ACM Workshop on Continuous Archival and Retrieval of Personal Experiences (CARPE-2004), Columbia University, New York.
Ark, W., Selker, T. (1999) A look at human interaction with pervasive computers. IBM Systems Journal, 38(4):504–507.
Balkenius, C., Moren, J. (2000)A computational model of context processing. Sixth International Conference on the Simulation of Adaptive Behaviour, The MIT Press, Cambridge, MA.
Buchholz, T., Kupper, A. (2003) Quality of context: What it is and why we need it. Workshop of the HP OpenView University Association 2003 (HPOVUA 2003), Geneva.
Bush, V. (1945) As we may think. Atlantic Monthly, 176(1):101–108.

Dey, A.K., Abowd, G.D. (1999) Towards a Better Understanding of Context and Context-Awareness, College of Computing, Georgia Institute of Technology, Atlanta GA, USA.

Anind, K.D. (2001) Understanding and using context. Personal and Ubiquitous Computing Journal, 5(1):pp. 4–7.

DiDuca, D., Van-Helvert, J. (2005) User experience of intelligent buildings: A user-centre research framework. IEEE International Workshop on Intelligent Environments, Colchester, UK.

Dourish, P. (2004) What we talk about when we talk about context. Personal and Ubiquitous Computing, 8(1):19–30.

Emerald Insight. (2009) http://www.emeraldinsight.com; last accessed February 2009.

Helal, S., Winkler, B., Lee, Ch., Kaddourah, Y., Ran, L., Giraldo, C., Mann, W. (2003) Enabling location-aware pervasive computing applications for the elderly. Proceedings of PerCom 2003 – 1st IEEE Conference on Pervasive Computing, Fort Worth, Texas.

Helander, J. (2005) Exploiting context histories in setting up an E-Home. 1st International Workshop on Exploiting Context Histories in Smart Environments (ECHISE-2005), Munich, Germany.

Huebscher, M.C., McCann., J.A. (2005) Adaptive middleware for context-aware applications in smart-homes. 2nd Workshop on Middleware for Pervasive and Ad-Hoc Computing (MPAC), Grenoble, France.

Loeser, A.F. (2003) Naumann: Semantic overlay clusters within super-peer networks. International Workshop on Databases, Information Systems and Peer-to-Peer Computing (DBISP2P), Berlin, Germany.

Mayrhofer, R., Radi, H., Ferscha, A. (2003) Recognizing and Predicting Context by Learning from User Behaviour, Austrian Computer Society (OCG).

Mulvenna, M.D., Zambonelli, F. (2005) Knowledge networks: The nervous system of an autonomic communication infrastructure. 2nd IFIP TC6 International Workshop on Autonomic Communication (WAC 2005), Vouliagmeni, Athens, Greece.

Nurmi, P., Martin, M., Flanagan, J.A. (2005) Enabling proactiveness through context prediction. Proceedings of the Workshop on Context Awareness for Proactive Systems, Helsinki.

Pentland, A. (2005) Socially aware computation and communication. Computer, 38(3): 33–40.

Petzold, J., Bagci, F. (2003) Global and local state context prediction. Artificial Intelligence in Mobile Systems 2003 (AIMS 2003) in Conjunction with the Fifth International Conference on Ubiquitous Computing, Seattle, USA.

Schilit, B.N., Adams, N., Gold, R., Tso, M.M., Want, R. (1994) Context-aware computing applications. IEEE Workshop on Mobile Computing Systems and Applications, Santa Cruz, California, USA.

Schneider, M., Bauer, M., Kröner, A. (2005) Building a personal memory for situated user support. 1st International Workshop on Exploiting Context Histories in Smart Environments (ECHISE-2005), Munich, Germany.

Sterritt, R., Mulvenna, M.D., Lawrynowicz, A. (2005) Dynamic and contextualised behavioural knowledge in autonomic communications. First International IFIP Workshop WAC 2004, Springer-Verlag, Lecture Notes in Computing Science, Berlin.

Strang, T., Linnhoff-Popien, C. (2004) A context modeling survey. Workshop on Advanced Context Modelling, Reasoning and Management as Part of Ubiquities Computing – The Sixth International Conference on Ubiquitous Computing, Nottingham, England.

Suchman, L. (1987) Plans and Situated Actions: The Problem of Human-Machine Communication. Cambridge University Press, Cambridge, UK.

Weiser, M. (September 1991) The computer for the 21st century. Scientific American, 265(3): 94–104.

Wilson, D.H., Wyatt, D., Philipose, M. (2005) Using context history for data collection in the home. First International Workshop on Exploiting Context Histories in Smart Environments (ECHISE), Munich, Germany.

Chapter 10
Prototyping Cognitive Prosthetics for People with Dementia

Richard Davies, Chris D. Nugent, and Mark Donnelly

Abstract In the COGKNOW project, a cognitive prosthetic has been developed through the application of Information and Communication Technology (ICT)-based services to address the unmet needs and demands of persons with dementia. The primary aim of the developed solution was to offer guidance with conducting everyday activities for persons with dementia. To encourage a user-centred design process, a three-phased methodology was introduced to facilitate cyclical prototype development. At each phase, user input was used to guide the future development. As a prerequisite to the first phase of development, user requirements were gathered to identify a small set of functional requirements from which a number of services were identified. Following implementation of these initial services, the prototype was evaluated on a cohort of users and, through observing their experiences and recording their feedback, the design was refined and the prototype redeveloped to include a number of additional services in the second phase. The current chapter provides an overview of the services designed and developed in the first two phases.

10.1 Introduction

Dementia is a chronic and disabling disease that affects the brain and exhibits typical symptoms including impairment of memory, thought perception, speech and reasoning. In an increasingly elderly population, concerns regarding the long-term care and support of such persons have emerged as a major issue, which warrants considerable investigation. One potential solution lies in the provision of ICT-based solutions. Indeed, a wide range of assistive technologies have been developed to support our ageing population, however, few of these technologies have specifically focused on

R. Davies (✉)
Computer Science Research Institute and School of Computing and Mathematics, University of Ulster, Jordanstown, UK
e-mail: rj.davies@ulster.ac.uk

M.D. Mulvenna, C.D. Nugent (eds.), *Supporting People with Dementia Using Pervasive Health Technologies*, Advanced Information and Knowledge Processing, DOI 10.1007/978-1-84882-551-2_10, © Springer-Verlag London Limited 2010

developing cognitive prosthetics for persons with dementia (Lauriks et al. 2007). Of the few studies conducted, one reported the use of electronic memory aids to assist persons with dementia to complete time-critical tasks such as medication compliance (Holthe et al. 1999). Another study reported the use of a simplified mobile utilizing a single button to facilitate a direct answering service (Kort 2005) and another reported on the use of televisits utilising video phones (Savenstedt et al. 2003; Mickus and Luz 2002). Both of these approaches were shown to have a positive effect on social communication. An important concern for caregivers is the area of safety; one study developed a system that could be used to monitor the location of a person with dementia by "tagging" their clothing and defining a safe zone, outside which an alarm is raised (Miskelly 2004). Although a number of these systems already exist and have been tested on persons with dementia, it is clear that there is no concise unified approach on how best to present a range of services to someone with dementia. The aim of the COGKNOW project is to try to address this issue by developing a user validated system that is both scalable and interoperable. To facilitate this scalability, off-the-shelf technology has been employed to permit rapid development and refinement. The project has identified four areas of cognitive reinforcement as previously presented in Chapter 4; support in these areas has been offered through the development of different services. The four areas investigated are as follows:

- Remembering
- Social communication
- Supporting daily activities
- Safety

In addition to identifying the four areas requiring support a patient inclusion criterion (see Chapter 4) was put in place and the service targeted for this cohort was based on their cognitive abilities. Only those persons diagnosed with mild-stage dementia according to tests such as the Mini Mental State Examination were invited to participate in the user trials. The identification of the four key areas and the inclusion of a specific cohort of users laid the foundation for a solid base from which key services could be identified and established. The following sections detail the services developed in the first two phases which have resulted in the realisation of the current cognitive prosthetic.

10.2 Initial Requirements

Prior to the first phase of technical development, a literature review was conducted to ascertain a small set of initial functional requirements which could be viewed as addressing the four key areas as previously mentioned. Having this small group of services in place allowed the first phase of the development to focus on the primary aim of evaluating the underlying technology for usefulness and user friendless.

Readers should make reference to Chapter 7 for more details on the user requirements approach used to generate the initial list of services. The initial list of services which were identified is outlined below:

- Basic reminding service
- Picture dialling
- Music service
- Door warning service

10.3 System Design and Components

The system design was primarily based around creating independent care for persons with mild dementia who were living at home either on their own or with their spouse. Through analysis of the initial requirements, four main system components were identified as being required to facilitate the initial services being developed: a table top touch screen display with accompanying processor, a mobile phone with touch-sensitive display, a server and a home sensor network. Three stakeholders exist in the system: the person with dementia, their primary caregiver and an informal caregiver or a healthcare professional. Figure 10.1 presents each of the four system components and highlights the roles of the stakeholders. Also presented are the interconnections that are required to support communication between the system components.

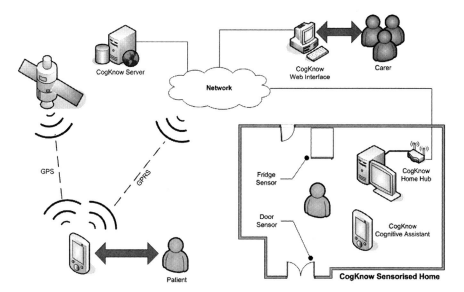

Fig. 10.1 System infrastructure highlighting major components and identifying stakeholders

In the following sections, an introductory description of each of the major technical components is provided in relation to their role within the system.

10.4 Stationary Device

The stationary device comprises of two primary parts, the first is a touch screen display and the second is a processor unit. The touch screen display provides an interactive mechanism through which the services can be offered to the person with dementia. The purpose of the processor unit is to act as the central hub inside the home environment, storing local data and relaying information to and from the central server. In terms of service delivery, the stationary device can be seen as the primary provider to the user. The stationary device has two main communication channels: the first is a local network which is supported by two wireless technologies: wi-fi for communication within the home environment and a proprietary RF channel for gathering data from the sensor network. The second channel is the main back bone to the system and connects the stationary device to the central server; this channel is supported by various Internet broadband communication technologies, for example, DSL and 3G.

10.5 Mobile Device

The mobile device offers the person with dementia the ability to access services inside and outside of the home environment; however, its main purpose is to provide assistance outside of the safety and familiarity of the home environment. The mobile device is a small lightweight device with a sensitive touch screen display capable of emulating services provided by the larger stationary component. One particular drawback of using the mobile device is the screen size which can only display a limited amount of information/services to the user. The mobile device has two modes of communication depending upon the context under which it is being used. The first is a local wi-fi network which is used when the mobile device is used inside the home environment. The mobile device channels all communication through the stationary device via the wi-fi network. When used outside of the home the mobile devices switches to 3G or GPRS (depending on service availability) and in theory channels all communication through the central server.

10.6 Sensor Network

The sensor network is a pervasive system that consists of a number of different sensor technologies that are strategically placed throughout the home environment. In general, the sensor network consists of two types: sensors and actuators. The sensors are based on a proprietary RF communication channel and have a small form factor approximately similar in dimension to a matchbox. Sensors are capable of detecting various events such as the opening and closing of doors. The actuator technology is based on a wired technology called X10 and uses the internal wiring infrastructure of the main power network to transmit data. Using X10 actuator technology, it is possible to control the state of various appliances throughout the home environment such as lamps and televisions.

10.7 Server

The server consists of a backend processing station that contains a central database and is the only major component which has a fixed location outside of the home environment. Its primary purpose is to hold all the information generated at a system level and organise this information in a meaningful and easily accessible manner.

In addition to the aforementioned major technical components a software infrastructure was designed to accommodate the provision of a range of services. The primary software component on the stationary device is Java based with smaller software components present to handle communication and XML handling. Figure 10.2 shows the various software layers in place to support and manage the range of services on the stationary device.

Fig. 10.2 Software infrastructure on the stationary device

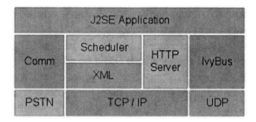

Having provided a brief description of the four major technical components and the software, Section 10.8 will focus more on the first and second phases of developments and present the various services that were deployed in each of the phases as a direct result of the development.

10.8 Methodology

A three-phase waterfall methodology was followed which consisted of three development and evaluation stages with each of the evaluation stages feeding into the subsequent development phase as shown in Fig. 10.3.

A small multidisciplinary working group within the Project Consortium was established with the main objective of composing the initial list of functional requirements as the entry point for the first phase of development. These functional requirements were spread across the four key areas of cognitive reinforcement,

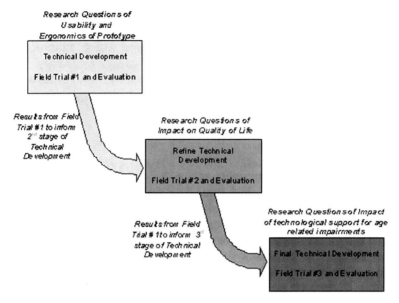

Fig. 10.3 Three-phased waterfall approach adopted as the basis of the methodology for the project

namely remembering, social communication and daily activities. To facilitate the rapid development process meant for the first phase, the initial set of functional requirements were limited to 12 in total. The primary concern was to have a basic system in place, which could be evaluated in terms of its usefulness and usability. Furthermore, a "top four" set of functional requirements were identified and initially focused upon to ensure that at least one service from each of the four areas of support would be developed. The top four functional requirements in ranked order of priority were a basic reminding service, a picture dialling service, a music service and a basic warning service for the front door being left ajar.

The first prototype was then evaluated on a group of 16 persons across three sites in Europe. The first field test focused on evaluating the technology to help ascertain its usefulness and user friendless. As the expected evaluation outcomes were basic due to the service provided, the duration of the field test was limited to 1 day. The first field test was supported at each of the three sites by research nurses and a technical researcher who were present to act in a supervisory role. Each of the services provided by the system was demonstrated to both the person with dementia and their caregiver. Following this a series of prescribed tasks were completed by the person with dementia and observed, from a clinical perspective, by the research nurses and at a more technical level, by the technical researcher. At the end of the field test semi-structured interviews were conducted on a separate basis with both the person with dementia and their carer. All observations and interview responses were recorded for future analysis to serve as valuable input to the second phase of the project. The above process was then repeated for the second phase of the development with the primary differences being the addition of new services and the refinement of existing services alongside an extended period of testing in the region of 1 week. At the time of writing this chapter, the project was in the middle of its third development phase. The remainder of this chapter will focus on the services that were created as part of the first and second phases of the COGKNOW project.

10.9 Services

The range of services offered to the person with dementia to help them navigate through their day were in general equally spread across the four areas of cognitive reinforcement:

- Remembering
- Social communication
- Supporting daily activities
- Safety

The services which span these four areas were supported in the first instance on the stationary device through touch screen technology to first convey information and second retrieve any interactions with the person with dementia. Before the following sections focus on each of the functional requirements in more detail Figs. 10.4, 10.5 and 10.6 illustrate the three different generations of the stationary device interface. It can be seen by comparing the first generation shown in Fig. 10.4 with that of the second and third (Figs. 10.5 and 10.6, respectively) that there have been significant changes regarding the look and feel and graphical layout of the stationary device.

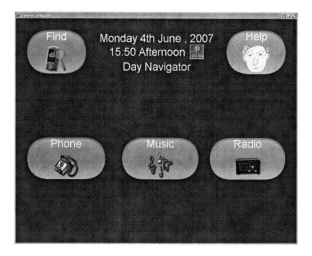

Fig. 10.4 First-generation stationary device interface

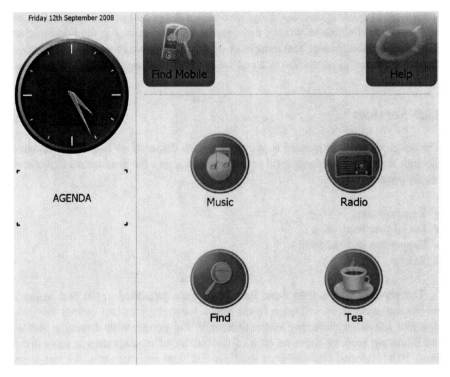

Fig. 10.5 Second-generation stationary device interface

A general theme across all three versions on the stationary device is that it consists of three main areas. These are emergency services generally located towards the top portion of the screen. The other areas contain the main list of services and those services related to time and reminders. All versions reserve the middle portion of the screen to activate services such as reminders and additional services that require subsequent actions after initial selection.

10.9.1 Remembering

The most important of these is remembering, which has been identified through the literature review as the main area of unmet user needs. To address this area a number of services have been developed. The primary service aims to deliver a series of on-screen reminders that contain personalised multimedia content to facilitate the person with dementia in performing a particular activity. The reminding service is a core service and is distributed across all four major system components. The server is responsible for the storing and configuration of reminders via a web-based interface that is targeted for use by the caregiver. Each reminder can be personalised in terms of the content presented to the person with dementia. The reminding service

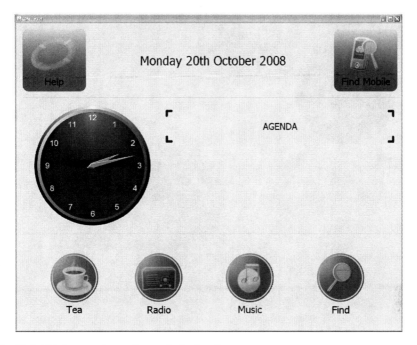

Fig. 10.6 Third-generation stationary device interface

supports configuration of various message types such as text, image, audio or video. Once a reminder is delivered to the stationary component it is queued and ultimately scheduled for delivery 2 min before its presentation to the person with dementia. When a reminder fires it is immediately presented to the user (Fig. 10.7) for a pre-defined period of 4 min or until the user acknowledges receipt of the reminder by pressing the reminder area on the touch screen.

In its current form the reminder service logs various pieces of information including whether the screen was pressed in acknowledgment of the reminder. In the third iteration of the system it is expected that the reminder service should support some form of real-time messaging system such as SMS to inform caregivers of a user's adherence to their reminder schedule.

In addition it is planned that the third development stage will have more control and configuration over the number of repetitions a reminder will make until it is removed by the system.

In addition to being supported on the stationary device the reminder service is also available on the mobile device at a more secondary level. Due to the limited screen size, processing ability and issues surrounding conversion of video formats the mobile device was limited to showing text and images.

Still under the umbrella of remembering, a date/time indication service has been created on both the stationary and mobile components to help persons with dementia orientate themselves during the day. The date and time are displayed to the user

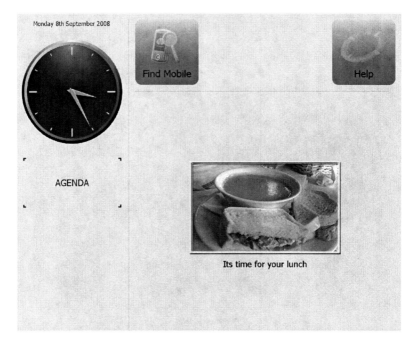

Fig. 10.7 An example "lunch" reminder on the stationary device

in country specific formats to support the deployment of the cognitive prosthetic at the three trial sites, namely the United Kingdom, The Netherlands and Sweden. The time component can be configured as either a digital or analogue clock. Additional personalisation can be made through the selection of a 24- or 12-h format, the presence of a "seconds" hand and the text size used to convey the date. Figure 10.8a and

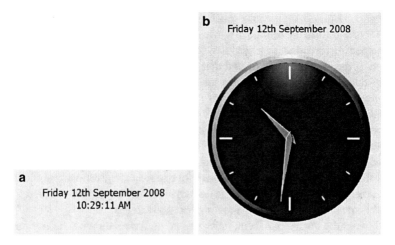

Fig. 10.8 a. Analogue time/date service b. Digital time/date service

8b shows the time/date component configured in both analogue and digital formats for the stationary component.

To complement the reminder service, an agenda service was developed on the stationary device to display a maximum of three prospective reminders. Each individual prospective reminder holds a short-textual description, the time of reminder delivery and a visual depiction of the time remaining until reminder delivery. There are two options available when configuring the visual depiction of the time remaining on a reminder. The time remaining can either be displayed as a circle divided into four quadrants (each full quadrant represents 15 min) or, as signal strength indicator formed by four decreasing levels (Fig. 10.9a and 9b). As the countdown to the reminder delivery continues the visual display changes the colour from green to red. An additional filter mode was implemented as part of this service to allow either all reminders to be passed onto the agenda service or when enabled the filter would only allow reminders related to appointments.

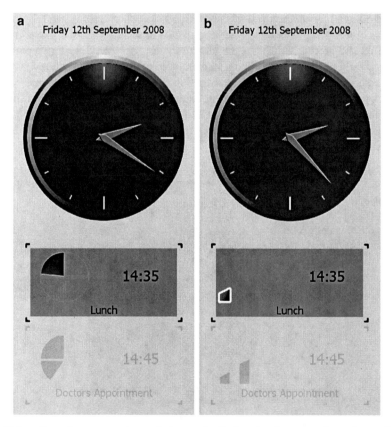

Fig. 10.9 a. Up to three prospective reminders can be displayed to the user on the stationary device b. A visual component is used to indicate the time remaining until the reminder is scheduled to be delivered on the main section of the screen

10.9.2 Communication

Social communication plays an important role for persons with dementia in helping to ensure that they can remain in close contact with their family members, friends and the local community. The literature supports the notion that using technology to support social communication can have positive social experiences and greater self-esteem in persons with dementia [3]. To help address this important cognitive area a picture dialling service has been developed. In the first phase, the picture dialling service was activated by pressing its related icon on the main menu, which then presented a list of contacts. To place a call, the person with dementia would have to carry out two more steps to complete the process. Performed in an arbitrary fashion these were lifting the phone handset and selecting a particular contact to call. Following user feedback, the second phase of development refined this service by reducing the number of steps required to place a phone call. This reduction in complexity was established by monitoring the on/off-hook state on the phone handset and allowed for the removal of the service's activation step. Instead, by using a wireless on/off-hook sensor the system was able to detect when the phone handset was lifted and promptly displays the picture dialling service. Selecting a particular contact would be the only additional step required to complete the call resulting in a two-step process yielding a one-step reduction from the previous phase one version. A photograph of the phone handset highlighting how it is mounted onto the side of the touch screen is presented in Fig. 10.10. Although not shown in Fig. 10.10 it should be noted that the handset has no keys for number entry and that all dialling control is offset onto the touch screen.

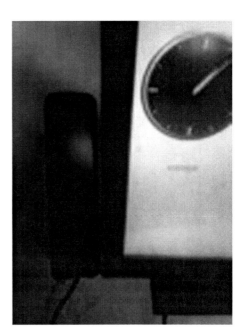

Fig. 10.10 Phone handset mounted onto the side of the touch screen

Figures 10.11 and 10.12 show the first- and second-generation picture dialling service both configured for four contacts, respectively.

An emulation of this service is available on the mobile device which is predominately for use outside of the home environment.

Fig. 10.11 First-generation picture dialling service

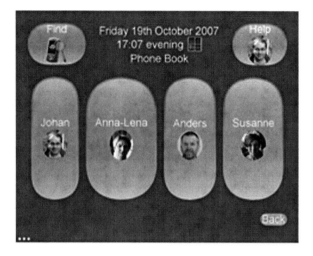

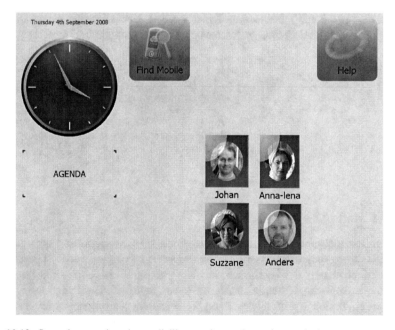

Fig. 10.12 Second-generation picture dialling service on the stationary device

10.9.3 Daily Activities

The range of activities that a person with dementia require assistance can be quite diverse. Identifying a common set of daily activities across cultural differences throughout Europe and inter-subject personal needs can also be quite difficult. Given the complexity that catering for various types of daily activities adds to the system a small set of services that were considered to be quite general were selected for development. The first was a very simplistic music playback service while the second was a more elaborate service to offer motivation through the eating process. In addition to these two fixed activities a general activity assistance service, which has the ability to offer assistance to the person with dementia when carrying out instrumental activities, was also developed.

10.9.3.1 Listening to Music

One common activity among the elderly in the home is listening to some music. Using current technology that can offer music playback becomes over complicated for persons with dementia hence the requirement for this simplistic service. The music service is simplified to consist of a single button on the touch screen, which resides in the main menu next to other services. Once pressed the button grows in size and becomes highlighted to indicate that it is currently active (Fig. 10.13). When activated the stationary device plays through a list of pre-selected favourite music in a random fashion. By pressing the button again the service is toggled to the off state that shrinks the button back to its original size and removes the highlight. The service name and icon used to depict a music service can be personalised to help the person with dementia feel more comfortable with the interface.

Fig. 10.13 Music service showing both (a) on and (b) off states

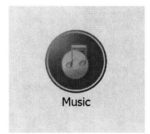 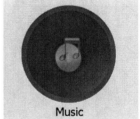

10.9.3.2 Motivation Towards Eating

Through the literature review it has been identified that supporting persons with dementia during the eating process can be supported by playing music (Yasuda et al. 2006). To adequately deliver this service the system must have the ability to detect when the person with dementia has started to eat. Sensor data obtained from within the home environment are analysed in real time and are controlled by a set of context rules which govern the detection of the eating process. The basic context rule that was put in place to achieve this was that the person with dementia is in the kitchen, it is lunchtime (predefined for each person), the fridge is opened, the oven is used and, finally, the person with dementia is sitting at the table. Once this sequence of events has been completed the system responds by playing music. The sensors put in place to help fulfil this contextual rule are as follows:

- Infrared movement sensor in the kitchen
- Software schedule sensor to detect lunchtime
- Open/close magnet sensor on the fridge and oven doors
- A pressure sensor on the chair at the kitchen table.

In the majority of installation processes the stationary device was located in a separate room to the kitchen such as the living room. Obviously this has implications in terms of facilitating the motivation to eat service through the delivery of audible music. To address this issue a set of wireless Bluetooth speakers were integrated into the system, which could be located at a suitable location to allow for optimum service delivery.

10.9.3.3 Assistance with Activities

To assist in activities that the person with dementia would otherwise find difficult to complete an activity assistance service has been developed. Due to the complexity involved in such a service initial development and testing were carried out in a separate development process to help minimise risk. Once the service had been identified as stable an integration process was completed to incorporate this as a main service on the stationary device. The activity assistance service operates by presenting a series of sequential video prompts about each step required to complete a particular task. In order for this service to be effective the video prompts must be recorded in the home of the person with dementia. The activity assistance service is flexible in terms of the number of steps and the types of activities it can support. A number of controls are provided on the screen to allow the person with dementia to skip to the next or previous steps, replay the current step or exit the service. Figure 10.14 shows how the stationary device may be installed to help give activity assistance support.

In some cases it may be difficult and/or dangerous for persons with dementia to try to operate household appliances such as lamps that may be inaccessible. An appliance control service was implemented to allow the user to control the power state of various appliances connected to the main supply network. A button to activate this service was presented to the user and could be personalised in terms of the text and associated image. Once the service was activated, the stationary device sent a control message using X10 technology via the power infrastructure in the home network using an X10 control module (left side in Fig. 10.15). An appliance module (right side in Fig. 10.15) intercepted the message and activated or deactivated the connected appliance accordingly.

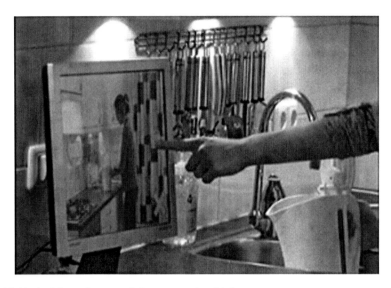

Fig. 10.14 Activity assistance to help prepare a hot drink

Fig. 10.15 X10 controller
and appliance module

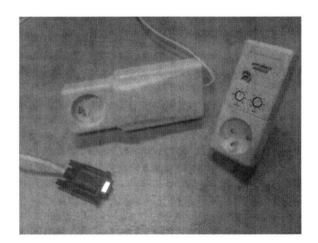

10.9.3.4 Safety

A primary concern especially for caregivers and family members of a person with dementia is their safety. There are two aspects that govern the safety of an individual with dementia. The first deals with safety within the home environment while the second aims to address safety issues outside of the home environment. High priority needs are that doors are closed and locked for security reasons and that assistance can be provided to navigate persons with dementia when they are outside of the home. In addition to providing assistance information to the person with dementia the system should also support the carergiver through provision of information about the status of the home environment and the location of the person with dementia. To help address these concerns and needs, a number of safety services have been identified to operate both inside and outside the home. The following sections describe in more detail each of the services that the system supports under the umbrella of safety.

10.9.3.5 Door Warning

A service that reminds people with dementia to close unintentionally ajar doors has been developed in the context of risk prevention relating to home security. Sensors located on both the front and back doors or any additional doors that provide access to the outside will monitor the open and closed state of the door. This service will trigger a reminder message after any door has been left ajar for a predefined period of time (Fig. 10.16). It operates two timer modes: one for during the day and a more time critical timer during the night due to the added security risk. The third-generation door warning service will aim to provide a "we-centric" service that could inform the carergiver about any security risks via SMS.

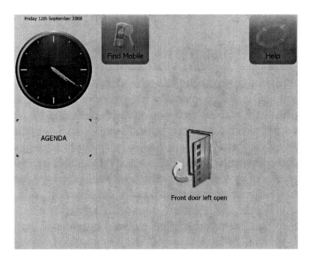

Fig. 10.16 Front door warning message

In order to provide additional safety-related services the door warning service can be cloned and reconfigured to offer a completely new service as other services can be based on the same technology. These include services such as warning about fridge and oven doors being left ajar for prolonged periods of time.

10.9.3.6 Emergency Contact

To help in situations where a person with dementia is in distress due to any number of safety factors, an emergency contact service which builds upon the picture dialling service has been developed. The main aim of this service is to enhance feelings of safety and to promote confidence in both the person with dementia and their caregiver. The emergency contact service is always visible and prominent to allow speedy access in moments of panic or stress (Figs. 10.4, 10.5 and 10.6). The primary concept behind this service is to eliminate the requirement for persons with dementia to remember or process information in order to arrive at a solution relating to who is the correct person to be calling. The service automatically calls the primary carer and in the third generation it is envisaged that if the primary carer is unavailable that a secondary and tertiary are contacted until finally calling a 24-h call centre.

10.9.3.7 Night-Time Wandering

Wandering during the night can cause a safety risk in relation to falls. To help address this issue a service is available that automatically activates a night stand light. This is achieved through the introduction of a bed-pressure sensor which can detect if the person with dementia has vacated the bed during the hours of darkness. When the person with dementia returns to bed the light is automatically switched off again.

10.10 Conclusions

A cognitive prosthetic has been developed which primarily consists of a stationary and mobile component present within a home environment. The aim of the prosthetic is to support persons with dementia by addressing four main areas of cognitive reinforcement: remembering, social communication, daily activities and safety. A three-phase methodology has been introduced to guide the development and refinement of the system based on valuable user feedback. To date, the first two phases of system development have been prototyped and evaluated. The third phase of development is currently under development taking into consideration the user experiences and technical issues arising from the previous two user trials. Over time, the cognitive prosthetic has matured in terms of the provision of its services, the system reliability and overall stability provided. Within each area of cognitive reinforcement the range of services have been developed, tested, evaluated and extended in order to improve and/or validate the approach that was adopted. The user-centred design approach coupled with a small notion of expert lead information proved to be a suitable approach in developing services for persons with mild dementia. Expert lead information was utilised whenever user-centred design information was either incomplete or provided inconclusive information. One of the main conclusions to draw from the prototyping process that was adopted is that it became obvious that a high degree of personalisation was required both across the system in terms of service selection and personalisation within each of the services. Ultimately this has led to the development of a dynamic set of services which have the ability to adapt according to a user's needs, wants and demands.

References

Lauriks, S., Reinersmann, A., van der Roest, H., Meiland, F.J.M., Davies, R.J., Moelaert, F., Mulvenna, M.D., Nugent, C.D., Dröes, R.M. (2007) Review of ICT-based services for identified unmet needs in people with dementia. Aging Research Reviews, 6(3):223–246.

Holthe, T., Hage, I., Bjorneby, S. (1999) What day is it today? Journal of Dementia Care, 7:26–27.

Kort, S. (2005) Mobile Coaching: A pilot study into the user-friendliness and effects of Mobile Coaching on the wellbeing of people with dementia and their informal caregivers. Faculty of Psychology, Vrije Universiteit, Amsterdam.

Savenstedt, S., Brulin, C., Sandman, P.O. (2003) Family members' narrated experiences of communicating via video-phone with patients withdementia staying at a nursing home. Journal of Telemedicine and Telecare, 9:216–220.

Mickus, M.A., Luz, C.C. (2002) Televisits: Sustaining long distance family relationships among institutionalized elders through technology. Aging and Mental Health, 6:387–396.

Miskelly, F. (2004) A novel system of electronic tagging in patients with dementia and wandering. Age and Ageing, 33:304–306.

Yasuda, K., Beckman, B., Yoneda, M., Yoneda, H., Iwamoto, A., Nakamura, T. (2006) Successful guidance by automatic output of music and verbal messages for daily behavioural disturbances of three individuals with dementia. Neuropsychological Rehabilitation, 16:66–82.

Chapter 11
ICT Interface Design for Ageing People and People with Dementia

Jonathan Wallace, Maurice D. Mulvenna, Suzanne Martin, Sharon Stephens, and William Burns

Abstract Ageing population trends, rising healthcare costs and social and digital inclusion are all factors in the background to the problem of older adults interacting with technology. Approaches to address "physical accessibility" and "access to technology" issues, as well as training for existing systems are evident, yet a usability issue still prevails. The primary aim of this chapter is to provide an overview of the research and literature and discuss the differing contexts in which older people and people with dementia interact with computerised systems and their associated issues.

11.1 Introduction

In Europe by 2050, it is estimated that one-third of Europe's population will be over 60. The number of "oldest old" aged 80+ is expected to grow by 180% (Eurostat 2002). For example, in 1951, there were 300 people aged 100 and over in the UK. By the year 2031, it is estimated that this figure could boom to 36,000 (BBC News 2007).

Governments are naturally concerned by these population trends, particularly with the associated rise in the cost of health care provision, due to the corresponding increase in chronic diseases such as diabetes, asthma, arthritis, heart failure, chronic obstructive pulmonary disease, dementia and a range of disabling neurological conditions. There are 700,000 people living with dementia in the UK today, a number forecast to double within a generation. Twenty-five million people, or 42% of the UK population, are affected by dementia through knowing a close friend or family member with the condition. One in three over 65 years will die with someform of dementia. (Alzheimer's Research Trust 2009). Indeed, the

J. Wallace (✉)
TRAIL Living Lab, School of Computing and Mathematics, Faculty of Computing and Engineering, University of Ulster, Jordanstown, UK
e-mail: jg.wallace@ulster.ac.uk

M.D. Mulvenna, C.D. Nugent (eds.), *Supporting People with Dementia Using Pervasive Health Technologies*, Advanced Information and Knowledge Processing, DOI 10.1007/978-1-84882-551-2_11, © Springer-Verlag London Limited 2010

World Health Organisation (WHO) has identified that such chronic conditions will be the leading cause of disability by 2020 and that, if not successfully managed, will become the most expensive problem for health care systems (World Health Organisation 2005).

However, charitable organisations are particularly concerned with the social factors, where this section of the population can find themselves increasingly excluded from society in a number of ways. In the report by the Digital Inclusion Panel (2004) aspects such as poverty, rural location and ethnicity were all cited as important factors contributing to exclusion from society. Initiatives have been trialled, which give free access to computer technology for the public at large. Public libraries have free access, for members, to the Internet. Access to technology is no longer a barrier to the older person as they are beginning to purchase their own PCs. A survey in 2003 found that "50% of people aged 60- to 64-years-old owned a computer with 37% online at home, and that they represented 12% of Internet users in the UK" (Jeffrey 2003). Indeed a recent survey by Hitwise a subsidiary of Experian in the UK has indicated that the aged 55+, the so-called silver surfers, are about to bypass the 35- to 44-year olds as the demographic age group representing the largest share of the UK Internet visits. Those aged 55+ represented 22.0% of the UK visits to all categories of websites in the 4 weeks to 12th May 2007, which was up 54% since 2005 and 40% since 2006. This compares to 23.5% of Internet visits from 35-to 44-year olds. It is interesting to note that this increase has come from both rich and poor alike. The Experian Mosaic classification allocates every household in the UK into 1 of 61 Types and 11 Groups. The Experian Mosaic groups Twilight Subsistence (pensioners subsisting on meagre incomes) and "grey perspectives" (pensioners enjoying retirement with savings to supplement their pensions) have both increased their online footprint. Internet visits from Twilight subsistence are up 29% over the past 2 years and visits from grey perspectives are up 30% (Hopkins 2007).

For the purposes of this chapter we utilise Ben Schneiderman's definition of the human–computer interface which takes into consideration the interface in its widest sense, not just with regard to screen design – "human–computer interface refers to the way a person experiences the computer, its application programmes, hardware components, output devices and functionality. It includes all aspects of the human's experience from the obvious ones of screen layout and selection options as well as input and output devices, reliability and accessibility." (Schneiderman 1996).

The older adult will be exposed to technological interfaces through necessity as technology moves on and becomes impossible to avoid. The increase in assistive devices in homes will also drive increased interaction with computer systems. The UK Government has become intent on moving towards a digitally inclusive society, measuring progress through results such as those cited in the 2004 report entitled "Enabling a digital UK" (Digital Inclusion Panel 2004) such as the finding that "five times more homes are connected to the Internet than in 1999" and "70% of government services are available online". For the purposes of the report Digital Inclusion is defined as "using technology as a channel to improve skills, to enhance quality of life, to drive education and to promote economic well being across all elements of society." (Digital Inclusion Panel 2004).

While physical accessibility has been addressed to some extent, there has been little or no attempt to rethink interface concepts to accommodate the older user and to reflect their specific problems with formation of suitable mental model for systems. The "Your Guide" system of free-standing public access kiosks was piloted in 2000–2001 by the UK Government and Consignia. This information kiosk was an effort to boost the flagging post offices and to help the UK Government deliver on its commitments to provide e-information to all (Keates and Clarkson 2003). Initially some physical requirements were identified which needed to be changed. Having been designed mostly by men, the pilot kiosks were generally too high for older women and others, to see the screen properly; the screen was too small to accommodate the larger size fonts needed for those with impaired vision. This resulted in only a few lines of text being displayed at one time. There was an increased need for scrolling, which had its own associated problems for the less agile fingers. The need to use both hands to operate the system was another obstacle, for those with walking difficulties, where one hand was needed to hold a walking stick or other walking aid. Lessons have been learned about physical limitation of older people but little attention has been paid to the other facets of decline due to natural ageing.

The functional needs of the older user also vary greatly from other sectors of users since most of the older users will not be using technology for business or work related tasks. They may wish to book cheap flights; after all they have more leisure time than the working population. They may see a greater need to communicate with family and friends across the world, e.g. sending e-mail to family members. Grandparents may be driven by the desire to see pictures or indeed video of a new grandchild, as a reason to access technology and overcome their initial fears. Fit older adults today will become progressively less able with age and many will live in a technologically supported living environment. The challenge for ubiquitous and pervasive computing in such supported living environments is in managing a sophisticated and dynamic perspective on computer-mediated interactions with human beings, without intruding unnecessarily into their lives. This is what is described as the notion of *calm* (Weiser 1991), where the computing resources quietly modify themselves to suit the needs of the user. An intuitive interface design would also be able to span different technologies and may be of use in the "Smart-Home" environment. This would in turn help to decrease healthcare costs, as more people would be enabled to live on longer their own.

Background research findings indicate that more research is needed to establish the main problems or obstacles that discourage older adults from using computerised facilities and systems. Few attempts have been made to redesign the interfaces with focused functionality and using more meaningful interface design to accommodate the older user. The primary emphasis to date has been on hardware issues, physical disability accessibility, web design and training for existing interfaces. A solution that enables a more intuitive information transfer between system and this user group could then be extended to span other user groups and various contexts of interaction. Many people over the age of 60 have difficulty using standard computer and communication devices. Even when the technology is made readily available to them, the uptake rate for making use of these facilities is poor. A technology rich

environment is becoming more and more commonplace and older members of society appear to have convinced themselves that they will never be able to cope with the
changes. Initially they are frightened and subsequently find the standard interfaces
of the devices confusing and difficult to understand. Not utilising this advantageous
technology is, not only decreasing the effectiveness of assisted living systems, but is
depriving older people of opportunities to improve their quality of life and reducing
their opportunity for social inclusion.

The remainder of this chapter is laid out in the following sections. In
Section 11.2, we present our overview of the research and literature grouped into
five areas:

- Age-related issues: targeting the issues raised for HCI and interface design in
  respect of physical and cognitive needs of the older population.
- Special requirements related to the user group: requirements beyond those of
  the physical needs of the older person, such as the diversity of the group and
  special difficulties in communicating requirements between the user group and
  the designer.
- Emerging approaches: new approaches to design for this user group.
- Broader technological perspective: other technological areas than the standard
  software and web applications – ubiquitous and pervasive systems as well as
  assistive technologies.
- Specific interface design issues for people with dementia.

Section 11.3 briefly discusses other associated issues and Section 11.4 presents a
discussion on the review findings and draws conclusions.

11.2 Ageing and Interface Design

Ian Stuart-Hamilton describes chronological age as an arbitrary figure since there
is no specific time when age happens (Stuart-Hamilton 1994). It is agreed amongst
professionals in gerontology that 60–65 is the "Threshold age" when the signs of
ageing become more distinct. Government too, tends to refer to those over 60 as
older adults. This may be because it is the age most people begin retirement and
have reduced activity. It is worth bearing in mind though that age is a natural, gradual
process and losses due to age can begin in early adulthood and only become more
obvious in the 60+ years.

According to Stuart-Hamilton (1994), ageing affects the sensory systems of the
older adult. Sight deficiencies include the loss of acuity (the ability to focus on
detail) especially in poor contrast or dim light. As vision deteriorates it becomes
more difficult for the eyes to recover from glare. Older people require a longer
time to process visual stimuli and also suffer from a narrowing of field of vision or
even loss of peripheral vision. Sight is not the only sense affected by age; hearing
is compromised too. Hearing losses include the loss of the ability to recognise
high-frequency sounds and the inability to distinguish the direction of source of a

sound. Hearing distortions are also more common with age; e.g. tinnitus, a ringing in the ears.

Other senses are affected by age but they do not have the same affect on intellectual skills as vision and hearing. Age deficiencies are more apparent when several functions must be used at once or when the message to the brain is a more complex message. Focusing of attention is diminished by age, and processes of the brain are generally slower (Stuart-Hamilton 1994). Since there is argument regarding exactly when ageing begins and the differences between young old and older old (which may have bearing on the service type the person wants to access and the mode that is most appropriate), for the purposes of this chapter we will define the use of the term older adult as persons aged 60–80.

The literature we have reviewed for this chapter although very varied in focus, facilitated a grouping into five broad categories:

- Age-related issues: targeting the issues raised for HCI and interface design in respect of physical and cognitive needs of the older population.
- Special requirements related to the user group: requirements beyond those of the physical needs of the older person, such as diversity of the group and special difficulties in communicating requirements between the user group and the designer.
- Emerging approaches: new approaches to design for this user group.
- Broader technological perspective: other technological areas than the standard software and web applications – ubiquitous and pervasive systems as well as assistive technologies.
- Specific interface design issues for people with dementia.

11.2.1 Age-Related Interface Issues

Many of the papers we have reviewed deal with the physical, psychological and other age-related issues which must be considered in interface design. While the usual guidelines of HCI (human–computer interaction) are to be applied, it should be considered which age-related issues apply and how HCI techniques can allow for these. Older adults are subject to changes in their intellectual skills in later life. The physical degradation and damage through age, to the Hippocampus especially, affects the ability to learn through exploration (Stuart-Hamilton 1994). This type of learning is associated with understanding computer interfaces, and is how the user understands the user interface for web and software applications. Older adults are still able to learn but in a different way, as discussed by Zajicek (2001). Zajicek looks at physical and other issues which affect interface design. Physical changes such as failing eyesight, diminishing intellectual skills and memory loss are the main issues which affect how a user interacts with a system. The memory loss associated with age means that the user is less able to cope with complex navigation structures or long lists of instructions. Care must be taken to reduce the load on the memory by using short messages, for example. Although learning is more difficult for the older person it is still possible. Different approaches to interface design should be used which result in interfaces which do not rely so heavily on exploratory investigation on the part of the user. Zajicek also points to the dynamic nature of the requirements for this user group. Tiredness and state of health or mind can have a significantly greater effect on the performance of these users when compared to other user groups. Grouping the users under the one term "older users" is misleading. It gives the impression of a homogenous group of people. Interestingly, a larger degree of diversity is found in this group than younger groups. Therefore the requirements cannot be regarded as a standard static set for all older users. One very interesting aspect that Zajicek points out is that although younger users and technophiles emphasise the convenience of computers and Internet as a main advantage, older users are not motivated by that argument. They may prefer a trip to the shop to talk to the shop keeper or to just get out of the house. This motivation can have a real influence on how well a person performs. Older people will accept technology but weigh up whether it is worth the effort; after all they may have to learn how to operate the keyboard before they master the Internet. Zajicek suggests that, to make systems and hence interfaces easier for older or sight restricted users, functionality should be reduced. While her suggestion is a valid one, it could be argued that a more universal approach to design might also be appropriate.

Hawthorn (2000) also discusses these age-related issues and the implications for HCI. Examining the factors, he agrees that because cognitive skills are affected by age, the load on the memory should be kept to a minimum. A simple, structured interface is important in order that all the cognitive powers can be concentrated on the task and not wasted on understanding the interface and the interaction process. His research suggests numerous tactics for increasing the usability of the interface through simple HCI techniques. His findings suggest that older users need greater contrast between text and background than other users (coloured text on coloured backgrounds slows the reader). He placed special emphasis on text size and recommended the use of simply structured layouts to increase clarity and consistency.

Investigations by van Horen et al. (2005) into instruction manuals also suggest some techniques to assist older people's comprehension of text and subsequent task performance. Older people require more time than average to read and digest text information, and they follow instructions better when they are segmented. He also emphasised, (because of short-term memory load restrictions), the importance of listing the most informative items first. Another important aspect he points out is feedback. A designer should always inform a reader what should happen or what he/she should expect to experience. These steps can improve task performance for the older user. Hawthorn also stresses the importance of target size. Large target size facilitates not only those with poor eyesight but also the less accurate mouse clicking reported with older users. Hawthorn makes some suggestions for design to facilitate those with impaired hearing. Lower sound frequencies are more appropriate for the older person. He has concluded, through this research, that even those with a high level of computer expertise will suffer from age-related barriers to continuing use of computers in later life. Expertise is generally restricted to a specialised field. As people age they experience difficulty in transferring their expertise to a new context. People currently approaching retirement age will have at least some exposure to computer systems. They will not necessarily be able to transfer their knowledge to a new system of the future. They will find it equally difficult to acquire the necessary new skills. The same age-related barriers to understanding a new system will exist, as for other older people, especially if the new system requires formation of a new mental model.

Feedback is an important facet of interface design and can play a significant role in error reduction and the visibility of a system, according to Norman (1992). Visibility is best explained by saying, "the better the visibility, the more obvious are the actions you need to take to achieve your goal." Feedback itself can be delivered using different modes, visual (sight), auditory (sound) and haptic (touch). Systems and interfaces use various types of feedback as part of their design.

Jacko et al. (2004) found that both novice and experienced older users can benefit from improved feedback combinations more significantly than the younger user groups. Although the experienced user performed well with drag and drop tasks, they also benefited from multimodal feedback. Their experiments used various combinations of haptic, visual and auditory modes of feedback. Their test groups included older and younger users of different computer experience levels. The results suggested that auditory feedback caused the greatest improvement in performance error reduction. Jacko recommends the inclusion of auditory feedback with or without any other feedback will prove beneficial in improving the manipulation accuracy of the older user. Their testing was using only a drag and drop scenario and further experimentation may be needed to prove the finding for other types of tasks.

11.2.2 Special Requirements Relating to Older People

In Zajicek's work, as discussed earlier, it was suggested that older people had different motivations for embracing technology. Systems may not have been explained to them in terms that they understood, and there were subsequent difficulties in forming a coherent mental model to aid understanding. This is not the only obstacle to "uptake" by the older population. Older people have a different perception to technology than younger adults, believing that it is not meant for them, or not of any use or relevance to them. Due to the distribution of wealth (Banks et al. 2006), which indicates that those with the most wealth are those aged 65–69 (i.e. retirement age) the financial barriers may not be as prohibitive as one might have thought. Attitudes to spending in younger generations and the current economic climate may also affect the distribution of wealth in future years. Technology is becoming more affordable, and free access is often provided in libraries and other centres.

Research by Patricia Wright et al. (2000) on text entry methods for handheld devices which included older users, suggests older people will accept new technology. As part of research to investigate whether users of different ages preferred on screen entry or keyboard entry of text, 50% of the older user group reported that they would use the PDA (Personal Digital Assistant), if they had won one in a competition. Wright's claims would tend to dispel the idea that older users will not engage with new technology.

Failing eyesight and motor skills are measurable physical effects of ageing, but it is evident from reviewing the research that simply enlarging text and minimizing functionality does not provide a complete and acceptable solution. The user group in question, i.e. the over 60s are not a homogenous group. They have different motivations and requirements beyond those which meet their physical needs. Time and life experiences lead this group to be the most diverse of all. Couple those distinctions with the complication of differing levels of computer expertise and it becomes clear that defining requirements for this user group is complicated.

According to Zajicek and Brewster (2004), participants at the 2002 HCI conference agreed that the "Dynamic Diversity" was one of the most important characteristics of the group. In the editorial they cite, amongst others, two important contributions to the research discussed at the conference, which have concentrated on the special difficulties encountered when dealing with older users: Eisma et al. (2004) and Lines and Hone (2004). Zajicek and Brewster conclude that a more sensitive and social approach is required and that the general design and data gathering methodologies must be adapted to be effective in this context. One important observation was that older people don't regard efficiency of performing a task as important as getting the task completed. The question of how to gather requirements from such a diverse group is examined.

The work of the researchers on the UTOPIA (Usable Technology for Older People – Inclusive and Appropriate) project, a collaborative research project amongst several Scottish universities, is discussed in a paper by Eisma et al. (2004). Their findings centre on how best to engage and deduce requirements from groups of older people and the disabled. They find that preconceptions are a major factor, old people might think they are too old to learn, or that they have no use for new technology. Since they don't have a clear understanding, having maybe never used any similar systems before, it is difficult for them to know what they require. It is also difficult for them to communicate what requirements they do have to, generally younger and technically minded designers. Usual methods must therefore be adapted for requirements gathering. Eisma et al. found that the social aspects of requirements-gathering encounters were very important. Loneliness, eagerness to please, fear of offending and cautious answers were all typical attitudes of the older adults involved in the UTOPIA research groups. The researchers tried various methods of requirements gathering. Focus groups proved difficult, if there were too many participants. Older people tended to stray from the discussion topic. When questionnaires were used it was found that the answers reflected a high level of non-committal responses. The recommendations were that focus groups should be kept small, questionnaires worded to force more commitment by the respondent and the use of hands-on examples and visual aids to increase understanding.

Lines and Hone (2004) also document the difficulties encountered in requirements gathering for this user group. The focus group method is generally recommended as an effective and cheap method of requirements gathering, used in this case to gather requirement regarding an IDAS (Interactive Domestic Alarm System).

It soon became clear to them that executing this method, as for other groups, had its difficulties. A focus group is intended to involve a large number of users at once to maximise time. This was unsuitable as too many participants only encouraged less useful discussion on the topic and more social interactions. Individual older people require a lot more attention and direction than the younger counterparts. The loose structure which is intended to promote free flowing ideas was too vague for the participants and it was found even semi-structured sessions had improved results. As a result they agree with Eisma et al. in suggesting the use of small highly structured focus group sessions. Where a deeper level of information is required individual interviews should be conducted. Any focus group conducted must only be done when the researcher himself has a clear understanding of the topic area, and can subsequently structure the session appropriately. This method would not be usable in an unknown domain. However the researchers, Lines and Hone, do not recommend completely excluding the older user from the process. It was evident from their findings that the older person still had a valuable input. The list of requirements provided by the carers of the users in the study, did not reflect the requirements that the older persons provided themselves. If those who have expertise and empathy with this group of people have difficulty defining requirements, how much more difficult is it for those who are primarily concerned with the technology to estimate appropriate requirements. It is clear that existing standard methods generally used must be adapted to gather appropriate user requirements.

Zajicek and Brewster refer to the study by Keates and Clarkson (2003) into the designing of an information kiosk for older users. They had found that 45% of the target user group could not use the first design of kiosk. This was due to mainly hardware issues, such as screen size, kiosk height and mobility issues. Once these physical issues were resolved, the interface itself also proved problematic. Use of inappropriate icons and inconsistent interface design paradigms caused difficulties for the older user in forming an appropriate mental model. They conclude that designers for older users must use some type of user-centred approach to design. The younger designer cannot design adequately for those outside his experience using standard methodologies. They also say that these users are the most likely not to conform to any standard user requirement assumptions.

During their research, Eisma et al. found Scottish businesses and industries to be uninterested in the older user group. Older people are currently a small part of the buying public and are less likely to buy new technology. Therefore they did not consider a business opportunity existed. Costs of specialist products are usually higher than mainstream products and so for systems to be available at a reasonable price they must have general appeal. A solution specific to one type of user has much less marketability than one generally accepted.

11.2.3 Emerging Approaches

Hawthorn (2003) agrees that the difficulty with making a system universally accessible is that simplification results in a system that no longer meets the required functionality of the experienced user. To satisfy a universal audience fully, a wide range of functions would be needed. To test the universal nature of "good design for older user" Hawthorn examines the design process of the previously developed "SeniorMail" system, an e-mail system developed specifically for a group of elderly users. He based his choice of which features to include and which to avoid primarily on literature research. He argues that other means of requirement gathering for such a wide diversity of user could not capture accurately the requirements. For example, general information on the range of "visual acuity" in the older population led him to the choice of font size, etc. Other features mirror those recommended in Hawthorn's earlier papers (2000), i.e. large targets, large buttons, colour schemes, simple navigation structure. He concludes that existing systems must be simplified to make them more usable for the elderly. He argues that it would be difficult to produce a system that would not exclude older users and yet remain attractive to younger more proficient users. While it may be possible to redesign web pages to accommodate a universal audience, this would not be able to be achieved in a programme software environment. Hawthorn concludes that universal appeal is difficult to achieve and that "senorised" versions of systems should be produced in the form of a simplified version of the real thing, which may be viewed as a training version of the full package.

A similar project "Cybrarian" (Dickinson et al. 2005) produced a specially designed e-mail system, rather than a redesign of the Windows version. The design included minimized functionality, accessibility features and simplified interface designs and structure. They also incorporated some features that the user could customize. Their conclusion is that they produced a system that was more usable (for the older user) than the standard packages available. They admit that more experienced users would need much greater functionality. In their design study, the design approach "Radically Simple", used in the development of the Cybrarian system, is discussed. Ironically the methodology is considered to create complexity itself as the designer attempts to increase any higher level of functionality. They suggest a layered approach may facilitate this. They admit these packages are usually marketed on increased functionality not less.

Both Hawthorn and those working on the Cybrarian project have noted the difficulties in the age gap between the designer and the older person. Even a middle-aged designer tends to make assumptions about older people which do not reflect the true requirements. Hawthorn insists that being informed of the difficulties is no substitute for first-hand experience (Hawthorn 2006). In her book *Ageing for Beginners* (Stott 1981) the author Mary Stott tells us ageing is relative in that no matter what age you are, you consider anyone 15-years-older as old. Regardless of what your age you still look out at the world through the same eyes and still feel the same person inside. Following this logic a 60-year old does not regard themselves as old and would consider someone aged 75 as old.

Gregor et al. (2002) concentrate on a different approach to deal with the diverse nature of the users and the dynamic nature of their requirements. They suggest an approach where, unlike the traditional method of seeking similarities amongst the users, the designer would seek out the differences. Since the user group is perhaps the most diverse they suggest that more research is required into structuring this approach. They also focus on the dynamic nature of the user requirements, the change over time, perhaps even over the span of the day or the changing environment of the user. It is suggested that, if this approach was to be taken, the resulting interface produced should be one that can accommodate the variety of needs and be adaptable to the situation and context. They also add that users should be able to personalise the interface. However, to allow personalisation of the interface can under certain circumstances also prove to be problematic. First if a service solution is designed for a SMART Home environment through which a district nurse or other professional care provider is able to monitor the patient in both the individuals' homes and remotely, then if personalisation/tailoring of the interface by the client is permitted, you automatically reduce the consistency of the interface for the professional carer across their case load, which as a consequence will cause increased search times and higher error rates when using the system in the individual clients' homes. This is the same reason behind large organisations insisting on having a common desktop environment to ensure consistency of the user interface across the organization. Second, with cognitive decline as a result of the onset of dementia, the end user will naturally become confused, and allowing continued personalisation of the interface for this type of end user, when they need more consistency not less, particularly with regard to colour usage and placement of navigation elements, will only add to their confusion.

The "User Sensitive Inclusive Design" (USID) methodology discussed by Gregor et al. claims that it may prove to be a useful approach to the problem. USID is suggested by Newell and Gregor (2000) as an extended form of User-Centred Design, where User-Centred Design is a common, standard approach to design in the HCI discipline. The original rationale of USID is based on the inclusion of disabled users, to help produce systems which can facilitate more universal access. It is referred to as sensitive rather than centred to reflect the diversity of the user group. It is difficult to represent the entire group completely. The inclusive nature of the design technique is emphasised to suggest that it is not possible to be truly universal, and they argue that universal design may not always be appropriate. This technique involves the designer attempting to facilitate all the possible users in the group. This will mean different approaches are required for requirements-gathering and other aspects of the design process.

11.2.4 A Broader Technology-Related Perspective

Up until 2003 most of the research and work in the topic area of design of interfaces for ageing people concentrated on Internet accessibility and web design (Hawthorn 2003), substantiated in the preliminary searches, which returned a high proportion of results regarding web design for older adults. Numerous guidelines and some legislation regarding the provision of accessibility to web sites for older and disabled adults are in place both in the UK and worldwide. Less work, however, has been done in the software and systems context, with regard to their interface design. Relentless advancements in technology have lead to advances in areas of *ubiquitous and pervasive computing* and heightened awareness in their application in the role of assistive technologies in the home context. These technologies will, in the very near future, be commonplace and whereas the active pursuit of purchasing technology may be avoided by elderly people today, the pervasive nature of these future developments will not be as easily avoided. When analogue television becomes obsolete, we will be forced to become users of digital TV. Currently, in the UK the Government is not only under pressure to fund state pensions for increasing numbers of retiring workers but also facing a healthcare financial crisis. Already care has been directed towards "in place" (in the home) solutions. The cost of care provision for persons living at home is a fraction of the cost of hospitalisation or institutional care. The 2001 Census revealed that there are approximately six million unpaid carers in the UK; these and other related statistics can be viewed at www.statistics.gov.uk. Consequently, ICT solutions are being sought.

It is reasonable to assume, as does Mynatt et al. (2004), that the general acceptance of sophisticated interface systems may stem from the development of a solution or integrated set of systems for the older user, and the need to facilitate independent living. They examine various technologies and their usefulness at Georgia Institute of Technology under the "Aware Home Research" initiative. In the Aware Home, technological support of the basic functions for living, referred to as ADLs (activities for daily Living) (Onn and Jin 1999), is the basis for the systems under investigation. They concentrate on three areas: overcoming the physical effects of ageing, the decline in cognitive ability (in particular loss of memory) and the support of the care network. With this and all of the discussed technologies, privacy, ethics and control are cited as concerns by the older people involved in this study.

The first generation of the assistive devices were primarily aimed at monitoring health and gave priority to the main preventable causes of elderly needing hospitalisation namely accidents and particular falls. Many homes have a now familiar alert system to call for help by activating a panic button. Falls are not only a common cause of death in older adults, but may bring on other conditions such as hypothermia or chest problems which cause death. Falls also cause a great deal of anxiety and fear after the event. People are afraid of falling again and so their normal life activities are affected. Those people who lay for an hour or more were 50% more likely to die within the next 12 months (McKenna et al. 2006). Blyth et al. (2005) challenge the focus of this first generation approach and call for "Socially Dependable Design". They suggest that the issue should be approached from a social aspect, incorporating social contacts and networks around the application of technology. They observe that much of the work done concentrates on the computer. While ergonomic design is an important facet and indeed requirement for universal inclusion, social facets such as improving quality of life should be addressed in the application of technology in the home of the older person. Through their research Blythe et al. draw attention to the evidence gathered in the interviews conducted which find that personal contact was very important to the older person. Their need for contact was demonstrated as false alarms, where the older person "accidentally" set off their alert button on a regular basis in order to talk to the warden of their fold or sheltered housing scheme. They also highlight that independence is viewed differently by the two groups of people involved, i.e. the health worker viewed the input device which calls for help as providing independence but the quoted statistics indicated that the older user viewed not wearing it as independence. While HCI can play a part in the design of the fall detection and monitoring systems that are expected to be widely available in the near future, HCI can also play a part in socially grounded systems. Attention is also drawn to the overarching issues of privacy, liability and freedom of choice, which are all valid and important issues that surround this topic area. The researchers argue that we may be in danger of attempting to off-load our responsibilities of care onto technological devices. Their "Net Neighbours" scheme is given as an example of "Socially Dependable Design". This socially dependable design paradigm depends on human volunteers; the statistics show the decline in voluntary work. They argue that systems which allow volunteers to give up smaller chunks of time and provide the service from, for example, their work area could be implemented.

While it is true many older people live alone, many also have a complex care system surrounding them. Different friends and family members, as well as official health care workers, may all be involved to a greater or lesser degree. This can be quite complex and in order for a carer to be productive he must ascertain what the current situation is, e.g. has the person had lunch yet? Did someone else wash sheets? The older person is the centre of such a network and so a system which helps co-ordinate care could help reduce strain on that older person is discussed by Consolvo et al. (2004). This research focuses primarily on the role of technology to assist the carers of the older person. It does suggest that pervasive technologies could play a major role in alleviating the stresses and miscommunication within the group of carers and the older person themselves; a system where the cognitive load of the older person is decreased. The issues of privacy and respect will become increasingly important as these new technologies advance from the first generation monitoring systems to those systems, which enable other access to the person's data, or perhaps vision-based sensing systems. The danger of systems controlling an older person's environment is the dependence the person may have on the technology and its reliability.

Ho et al. (2005) found in their studies that older people had less confidence in their own judgement and so were more reliant on the decisions made by the technology. They conclude that this trait in the older user must be factored into design. The older user is less likely to pick up on an error due to the software or the technology and would be more likely to blame themselves, if something was wrong. This could make them vulnerable if the context where this technology was used was a decision making system, e.g. monitoring medication intake.

Other researchers in the field look to technology in the home to help promote healthy behaviour, rather than a medical or environmental control system. Intille's research suggests using the emerging technologies of context-aware computing and mobile communication to create an atmosphere to encourage healthy behaviour patterns (Intille 2004). Work has already been done on projects that encourage walking activity and on those which provide information at what is called "the point of decision making" as a feature, which can aid those with memory impairment.

Perry et al. (2004) examine the Millennium Home system, and is set in the context of a healthy older user who may develop conditions later in life. The system employs multimodal interaction and aims, primarily, to provide "context sensitive" appropriate two-way communication that does not require the person to wear an input device. As discussed earlier the wearing of such a device can be viewed as a diminishment of the person's independence rather than the facilitator of independence as intended. Perry et al. base their theories regarding the design of interfaces for such systems on those of forerunners, who state that the interface is the crucial part of any such system. They suggest that as speech and vision are the most natural forms of communication these modes are therefore an obvious choice for user interfaces. They argue that "natural and context sensitive interaction" can be achieved by employing multimodal forms of interactions. They examine the interaction value of the different modes themselves and the trade-offs between them, e.g. auditory signals or instructions are only available temporarily so may be most appropriate for alarms or to draw attention (The home environment can be full of distractions.) Written text is there to be viewed for a longer period of time as an advantage to those with lower cognitive abilities. The mode of the interaction is also dependant on the type of content and form of information trying to be conveyed. They point out difficulties in incorporating various modalities in a design, mode-switching and mode-mapping; the various modes must follow the same rules, paths and expected sequences, etc. They also argue that mode switching can help allow for the dynamic nature of this user group's requirement. This may imply that this type of design is by default, attractive to all users and can promote universal inclusion. However they cannot substantiate their hopes that it allows for the entire diversity of the users group. The interactions took place via telephone (speech lists and button selection), TV/monitor screen (menu and remote control) and loudspeakers, sensors, voice recognition input. Interactions were designed on the basis of physical and activity context, urgency and interaction history, as well as allowing for physical limitations and general cognitive decline. The researchers had recognised the issues of intrusion and privacy, user control and had considered these in the design. This is not a system tested beyond the laboratory conditions of the Millennium Home itself. Introduction on a general scale would have many issues to be examined, such as security. Perry et al. suggest that if some intelligence were incorporated into the system it would allow for further functionality and an improved system.

Experimental research has been done by Bickmore et al. (2005) into relational agents. Defined as "computational artefacts designed to build and maintain long term social-emotional relationships with users", relational agents are the subject of research on the periphery of this topic area, concentrating on promoting healthy behaviours. They have studied the effects of using these agents to promote healthy habits amongst older people. The have found that the relationship built up between the person and the agent has better results when compared to non-relational systems. They argue that this facet of the system made it more acceptable to the older person and that it may be beneficial in motivation and in reducing loneliness for the older person, as well as nursing care contexts.

A similar design approach to Bickmore et al. is suggested by Forlizzi et al. (2004) by researchers in assistive robotics at Carnegie Mellon University. "Ethnographic Design Research Methods" are those that involve viewing the older person, the technology and their activities as a system to better understand the dynamics of the person's environment. The study of the relationship formed between the person and products and activities is a similar idea to that of the use of relational agents. Both are socially based. The researchers found that older people are more likely to only want a product that fulfils a functional need, they keep items which help them retain a sense of independence and dignity, and they rank social activities as high priorities. They suggest an "Ecological" design technique which incorporates the three aspects of person, product and activity that could produce a better product. They insist that social elements should be included in the design process.

Of course although the home becomes a more important focus for the older person (Stott 1981), there are other environments in which older people use technology and experience difficulties with the interaction. Earlier the *e-information* kiosk was discussed where elderly people could access information at the post office using the stand-alone kiosks. Many older people wish to drive their car for as long as possible; the car is a sign of independence for many sections of the population, not only older people. However, older people are finding the information displayed on the dashboard more difficult to interpret. The increased availability of navigation systems too can be difficult for elders to interpret. May et al.'s paper (2005) researches this problem. Based on the fact that cognitive decline has a detrimental affect on a person's ability to find their way through a strange environment, May et al. investigating the problems for older drivers, with the interface of in-car navigation systems. Their findings were that incorporating landmarks along side distance information had a positive effect on both confidence and accuracy, for the older driver particularly. Their findings support some of the work discussed earlier. The technology was accepted because of its functional benefits. Visual display was enhanced by another mode of interaction, i.e. auditory prompts (older people require longer to take in visual information) and less complex displays improved performance. They conclude that their inclusive design technique will improve the usability of the system for all users.

A "person centred technology evaluation" by Bagnall et al. (2006) reported that many of the participants considered themselves lonely, surprising since they lived in shared accommodation. They did not choose to be lonely; they had etiquettes and social rules which meant they would not want to disturb each other after 6 pm or when they had visitors. Bagnall et al. also focus on contexts where interaction with modern devices is difficult for the user. In particular they look at social contexts such as communication. E-mail was discussed earlier, but perhaps as a computer-based package rather than from its importance in social aspects of an older person's lifestyle. Mobile phones, chat rooms, gaming, etc. are all commonplace for younger users and yet many poor designs of hardware and software limit the accessibility of these social technologies for older users. This is particularly unfortunate since time and again throughout this review of the research and literature the work has all pointed to the increased need for social inclusion and the appreciation of the older population to social activities, as well as their acceptance of devices to facilitate this. The ethnographic research techniques employed by Bagnall et al. were introduced earlier in this review as a way of studying the needs of the older person through the study of the environment into which the system will fit. They studied the device's place in the home, the activity of contacting friends whether face-to-face or via other communication means, the timings associated with this and the system itself. They designed to overcome etiquette of older people and interface issues such as scrolling and sequencing of conversation. They designed a different type of computer gaming that did not involve the computer enforcing rules, etc. and noticed that the time spent socialising during the game was quite significant. They introduced an audio communication package to facilitate social interaction. They conclude, as do many of the previous papers, that the social requirements for elders are a very important part of the design process. They are a group that have a very different set of social interaction etiquettes from the younger generation.

11.2.5 Specific Interface Design Issues for People with Dementia

The loss of short-term memory in the elderly as a result of a cognitive disability, such as dementia, is a problem for the person and for their family and carers. Social activities and interactions become difficult, especially as their condition progresses, as these activities and interactions require a functioning short-term memory for effective participation.

Emerging technologies have the potential to play an important role in improving the quality of life for people with dementia. To achieve this potential the design and development of user interfaces, which very often act as a barrier to people with dementia, is overcome.

One of the biggest problems facing developers of assistive technologies for intended use by the elderly or those with a form of physical or cognitive impairment are issues relating to the usability of the user interface. This issue is further complicated by the largely differing needs exhibited by the end user along with the necessity of adaptation to generate a personalised, user-specific assistive environment (Hariz et al. 2007).

Today's technology features state of the art interface solutions, such as touch screens, styli and hand/voice recognition as well as standard WIMP (Windows Icon Menu Pointer) interfaces (Abrams et al. 1999). All of the aforementioned technologies potentially complicate the development of a user interface given the vast range of functionalities that they can support. For example, a WIMP interface on a touch screen monitor decreases the system's usability because the menu's hit area is so small and the user's finger is not as precise as a pointer.

Alm et al. (2004) states that computers can be used as a cognitive prosthesis, which can help augment human intellect. A cognitive prosthesis should provide a compensatory strategy for people with dementia which, when added to their environment, increases their ability to function (Alm et al. 2004).

11.2.5.1 Dementia in User-Centred Design

Despite the increasing number of dementia sufferers, it is still common that a range of research excludes this group (Savitch and Zaphiris 2005). There is, however, a growing recognition that people with dementia should participate in research; as such people with dementia are being included in the design, development and evaluation of the services they use. The methodology of this research should focus on the participant's strengths. The feasibility of some methods involved, such as storyboarding, should be considered. Stalker et al. (1999) states that questions themselves can be threatening to someone with cognitive impairment. Bamford (1998) also suggests that the following Table 11.1 should be taken into consideration:

Table 11.1 Considerations when interviewing people with dementia

1. Family carers and staff may feel the need to be present and this may confound the validity of response

2. People with cognitive impairments function best in familiar surroundings

3. People with cognitive impairments can most easily comment on their immediate surroundings

4. People with cognitive impairments may need the aid of stimulus materials to discuss abstractions

Researchers and interviewers should note that when asking someone with dementia a question, that it is not inconceivable that the person with dementia is concerned with giving the correct answer, when in actual fact there is no correct answer.

When considering the design and usability of a user interface for people with dementia, it is imperative to keep the interface distinctive, familiar and legible. This will enhance the feeling of familiarity that a person with dementia needs.

11.2.5.2 Previous Research for ICT and People with Dementia

There have been various studies undertaken to provide computer-based help for persons with dementia, these range from personalised web pages to interactive games or reminiscence scrapbooks. While these systems and services are widely available for people without a cognitive disability, the development and adaptation for persons with dementia remain a problem.

Alm et al. undertook a pilot study that presented people with dementia with a "Reminiscence Scrapbook". The aim was to determine what multimedia components would be best to present to the person with dementia. These included text, video, pictures and music/sound. The general finding of this study was that the multimedia presentation interested and motivated the persons with dementia. The feedback for the system was constructive and encouraging. Staff and carers were unable to identify anything they did not like, however one patient did say they did not like something about the system, but when questioned further they were unable to elaborate. Carers also believed that the choice of material prompted the patients to speak more than usual. In relation to the technology used, everyone found the use of the touch screen to be beneficial. One carer suggested that the option to customise the interface would be preferable (Alm et al. 2004).

11.2.5.3 Development of GUIs (Graphical User Interfaces) for People with Dementia

Before embarking on an entirely new concept for the design of interfaces for use with dementia, it is useful to consider established approaches to date. Although these may not be the end result for the target cohort, they should be considered to be generic enough to at least be considered as a starting point upon which further changes may be made.

One of the fundamental standards of interface design is that of psychologist Paul Fitts, commonly known as Fitts' Law. This states that the time taken to move from a starting point to the target depends on two factors: the distance to, and size of, the target (Fitts 1954). By following the principles of this law, designers are advised to make the clickable icon a reasonable size. Not only does this law help us determine the size of the icon, but also their position on screen. For example buttons positioned on the corners of the screen are more efficient because it reduces the possibility of the user overshooting the target (Hale 2007). Today's technologies have come a long way since the days of Paul Fitts. Fitts' Law provides us with an excellent approach in developing WIMP interfaces. Nevertheless, the time taken to move from a starting point to a target becomes irrelevant, if a touch screen or styli is used.

Another law is Hick's Law, which states that the time taken for a user to make a decision is determined by the number of choices they are presented with. The user does not consider each option one-by-one, but instead they sub-divide the options into categories. Users will make a quicker decision from a list of ten options than two lists of five. This law provides us with a good platform from which we can develop menu structures. Nevertheless, when developing interfaces for assistive technologies, we have to consider the disability of the end user. A cognitive disability, such as dementia, will mean the users may become confused if too many options are presented at once, however, if not enough options are presented then the user will have to burrow their way down through various different menus to reach the service they require (Burns et al. 2008).

When developing a system that will be in continuous daily use, it is imperative to include the end user throughout the technology development cycle and most importantly the GUI. If an end user cannot be relied upon to provide constructive feedback then a qualified professional should be consulted in conjunction with them. For example, if the system is for a patient with mild dementia, then their feedback may fluctuate. In this case their carer should be consulted.

11.3 Other Issues

Issues are raised such as privacy and confidentiality and the emotional needs of the older person in many, if not most, of the research papers reviewed for this chapter. Older adults are in a more vulnerable position than most, and their privacy must be respected. They must at all times be afforded the same rights as other user groups, and the tendency to treat them as one would treat a child must be avoided. Their personal details and medical records are confidential and must remain confidential. Systems that are put in place, to aid the daily living of the older adult, must ensure that they do not compromise the rights of the individual in the pursuit of a solution. The question of independence or perceived independence is also a major issue. It is important that older people feel their independence is not being diminished by a system. It is vital to the acceptance that the person remains in control of his environment.

11.4 Discussion and Conclusion

The material reviewed has naturally lent itself to be categorized into five areas that have been titled: age-related issues, special requirements of the user group, emerging approaches, a broader technology-related perspective and specific interface design issues for people with dementia.

With regard to the age-related issues the reviewed papers have dealt with the physical and psychological age-related issues that should be considered during interface design. Zajicek discusses the problems of failing eyesight, hearing and memory loss. She suggests that a different approach to interface design is required to mitigate for the older person's loss of investigative learning techniques. The motivations of the older person are examined, finding convenience to be less important to this user than to younger groups of users. Reduced functionality is her recommendation to simplify the human–computer interactions. Hawthorn and Van Horen concentrate on the physical age-related issues. Their suggestions are for simplified structure, contrast between text and background, increased text and target sizes. Van Horen also suggests segmentation and presentation of most informative information first. Julie Jacko et al.'s paper concentrates on feedback and the advantages of using multimodal feedback are discussed. Her findings suggest auditory feedback to be the most beneficial and Hawthorn recommends using lower frequency sounds for this user group. The papers in this section also suggest that experienced computer users will also suffer the same age-related issues as novice users.

With regard to the special requirements of the user group the reviewed papers discuss acceptance, diversity, appropriate mental model, information gathering difficulties and issues relating to older peoples' attitudes and etiquette. As part of her results in investigations involving the use of PDAs, Wright concludes that acceptance of technology by the older user is evident. The greater diversity of this group compared to younger user groups is highlighted by the work of Zajicek and Brewster. They also recommend the use of a more sensitive, social approach when interacting with the user and the need for the use of appropriate mental models. Eisma also found the need for a social approach to the user and highlights the difficulties in communications between user and the younger designer. Eisma also suggests use of carefully structured questionnaires to force committal from the user and to improve the quality of results. Eisma's main recommendation is for the use of small focus groups of approximately three users, or even one to one interviews during requirements gathering. This is reiterated in the work of Lines and Hone who also recommend small structured focus group work.

With regard to the emerging approaches, Hawthorn's paper recommends the reduction of functionality to accommodate the older person's needs. Dickinson et al. found that using a simplifying strategy in their approach to design caused difficulties and admitted that the resulting lack of functionality affected the acceptance of the product for more experienced users. Gregor et al.'s paper focuses on the need to design for the dynamic nature of the user requirements, changing perhaps daily or hourly. Gregor et al. suggest user-sensitive inclusive design, where USID is an adaptation to the standard User-Centred Design (UCD) approach which aims to seek diversity instead of similarity to promote inclusion.

From the broader technology-related perspective other technologies will impact in the daily life of the older person, whether they choose it or not, due to the increase in pervasive computing systems. Assistive living devices will become more commonplace especially in view of the ageing population and the associated healthcare burden. Mynatt et al. suggest that the trigger for more wide spread use of assistive devices may stem from their development for use in the area of elder healthcare. Blyth et al.'s paper suggests we are in danger of "off-loading" our responsibility for elder care to technology and we should use a socially dependable approach to design. Consolvo et al. focus on the role of technology in the care network of the elderly person. An investigation into the Millennium Home and context-aware computing features in the work of Perry et al., where they argue that multimodal forms of interaction are required in a context-sensitive environment. The researchers in the papers featured in this section also point out the overarching issues of privacy, security, liability and over-dependence. While most of these papers research home-based technology, May et al. examine improving the interaction of the older driver with the car-navigation system. They find evidence to support the suggestion that older people require longer to decipher information and suggest "Land marking" can aid understanding for all but especially the older users. Combining auditory prompts was also found to increase the usability. Forlizzi et al. apply an ethnographic approach when designing a product for the elderly. They argue that this approach can produce a better product as it involves studying the "ecology" of the person, the product placement and the activities involved. Bagnall et al. also used ethnographic research techniques to aid design of their system. They concluded that the social interaction facilitated by the system was as important a requirement as other more functional requirements. They also reported that the user group operates under a very different set of social rules and etiquette than younger user groups.

With regard to specific interface design issues for people with dementia, including persons with dementia to assist in guiding the development of assistive technologies is something that should be pursued to its fullest extent. This inclusion encourages the development of usable, familiar and tailored assistive technologies. Current strategies for user-centred design may be more focused on persons without a cognitive disability, however, work by Bamford and Stalker has provided a clearer methodology from which to carry out user-centred design with persons with dementia.

Technology can be used as a valuable tool for persons with dementia; however, the effectiveness of the technologies relies on the ability of the end user to use it. As mentioned above, the usability of the user interface is one of the major factors in the slow uptake of assistive technologies for persons with dementia. The current concepts of user interface design provide a sound basis from which to work from. However, these concepts should be tweaked and reworked to suit both the technologies and end user.

From the research it would appear that there are many valid age-related issues that affect the interaction of older people with technology. These are not only physical but also psychological and motivational issues that are directly due to age. These issues map to different aspects of the system and the interface. Physical issues have a direct relation to the physical elements of the interface, e.g. font size and contrast, while psychological and motivational issues have more bearing on the higher level design structures of the interface and the system functionality.

Some special requirements are not a physical symptom of ageing but are unique to this group. Many of the researchers have made mention of the wide diversity which exists within the user group and how the traditional methods of design do not cater for it and much of the basic understanding deficits reported in the research have been attributed to the user applying an incorrect mental model.

Generally we would accept that older people are quick to alienate themselves from technology, but research has shown that the group is not adverse from using new technology. Given the right motivation and circumstances the user group has proven keen to embrace emerging approaches in technology. One aspect that would seem to separate this group of users from all others is the great emphasis which is put on social factors. Perhaps it is because these users have trodden many paths, seen fads and fashions come and go and now have a deeper understanding of what is important in their lives, that they choose to prioritise social interaction above all else. This different approach itself can cause a barrier between them and the system designer. In the emerging approaches papers, some researchers approached the problem by reducing the functionality of present systems. They judged this to have limited success as experienced users of those systems were frustrated by the basic versions. Other emerging approaches concentrated on the treatment of the user rather than attempting to adapt an existing system. This treatment of the user called USID suggested different approaches and techniques for requirements gathering and other face-to-face time with the user group. The major shift towards designing for diversity rather than trying to find the common ground is also part of this approach.

Excluding a group of society from enjoying the benefits of technology is an issue of social inclusion. However, the problem is not restricted to computers and has wider implications. Elder healthcare could be delivered more efficiently and more cheaply if the problem could be overcome. The research involving applications in this area emphasises the importance of user involvement and the importance of allowing a person to remain in control of their environment. They call for socially aware computing for these users.

Some may argue that computer interaction will not be a problem for the elder person of the future, given their current exposure to technology, however, research has proven that even those who were considered to be computer literate experienced these difficulties. A solution to this problem will therefore not only help the older population of today but also the generations to come.

Acknowledgements The TRAIL (Technologies for Rurality, Ageing and Independent Living) lab represents the development of innovation and research thinking in Northern Ireland to support independent living across several key disciplines including business, information and communication technologies, occupational therapy, art, health care, social care and clinical medicine. Based at the University of Ulster, TRAIL is focused on supporting this diverse set of stakeholders as we develop new technologies, research perspectives, processes and integrated service solutions that deliver real value to our users, the ageing people in the North of Ireland and further a field across Europe.

References

Abrams, M., Phanoutiou, C., Batongbacal, A. et al. (1999) UIML: An appliance-independent XML user interface language. Computer Networks, 31(11):1695–1708.

Alm, N., Astell, A., Ellis, M., Dye, R., Gowans, G., Campbell, J. (2004) A cognitive prosthesis and communication support for people with dementia. Neuropsychological Rehabilitation, 14(1/2):117–134.

Alzheimer's Research Trust. (2009) http://www.alzheimers-research.org.uk/info/statistics, accessed 8 January 2009.

Bagnall, P., Onditi, V., Rouncefield, M., Sommerville, I. (May 2006) Older people, technology and design: A socio-technical approach. Gerontechnology, 5(1):46–50.

Bamford, C. (1998) Consulting people with dementia. Cash Care, Spring, 2.

Banks, J., Smith, Z., Wakefield, M. (2006) The Distribution of Financial Wealth in the UK: Evidence from 2000 BHPS Data, p. 11. Available at: www2.warwick.ac.uk, accessed on 5 December 2006.

BBC News (2007) Source: http://news.bbc.co.uk/1/hi/health/395143.stm, Accessed 27 March 2007.

Bickmore, T.W., Caruso, L., Clough-Gorr, K., Heeren, T. (2005) 'It's just like talking to a friend' relational agents for older users. Interacting with Computers, 17:711–735.

Blyth, M., Monk, A.F., Doughty, K. (2005) Socially dependable design: The challenge of ageing population for HCI. Interacting with Computers, 17:672–689.

Burns, W., Nugent, C., McCullagh, P., Zheng, H., Finlay, D., Davies, R., Donnelly, M., Black, N. (2008) Personalisation and configuration of assistive technologies. Engineering in Medicine and Biology Society, 30th International Conference of the IEEE, 20–25 August, pp. 3304–3307.

Consolvo, S., Roessler, P., Shelton, B.E., LaMarca, A., Schilit, B., Bly, S. (2004) Technology for care networks of elders. IEEE Pervasive Computing, 3(2):22–29.

Dickinson, A., Newell, A.F., Smith, M.J., Hill, R.L. (2005) Introducing the Internet to the over – 60s: Developing an e-mail system for older novice computer users. Interacting with Computers, 17:621–642.

Digital Inclusion Panel. (2004) Enabling a Digitally United Kingdom, a Framework for Action. The Cabinet Office, London. http://www.cabinetoffice.gov.uk/publications/reports/digital/digitalframe.pdf Accessed 18 October 2006.

Eisma, R., Dickinson, A., Goodman, J., Syme, A., Tiwari, L., Newell, A.F. (2004) Early user involvement in the development of information technology-related products for older people. Universal Access in the Information Society, 3:131–140.

Eurostat. (2002) NewCronos Database (Health and Safety), statistics – Key Data on Health 2002. Eurostat Morbidity Seminar, London.

Fitts, P.M. (1954) The information capacity of the human motor system in controlling the amplitude of movement. Journal of Experimental Psychology, 47(6):381–391.

Forlizzi, J., DiSalvo, C., Gemperle, F. (2004) Assistive robotics and ecology of elders living independently in their own homes. Human Computer Interaction, 19:25–29.

Gregor, P., Newell, A.F., Zajicek, M., 2002, Designing for dynamic diversity – Interfaces for older people. ACM SIGACCESS Conference on Assistive Technologies, Proceedings of the Fifth International ACM Conference on Assistive Technologies, Solutions for Aging, pp. 151–156.

Hale, K. (2007) Visualizing Fitt's Law, October 3rd, 2007; http://particletree.com/features/visualizing-fittss-law Accessed 2 November 2008.

Hariz, M., Renouard, S., Mokhtari, M. (2007) Designing multimodal interaction for assistive robotic arm. IEEE 10th International Conference on Rehabilitation Robotics, Noordwijk, The Netherlands.

Hawthorn, D. (2000) Possible implications of ageing for interface designers. Interacting with Computers, 12:507–528.

Hawthorn, D. (2003) How Universal is Good Design for Older Users. CUU 2003 November 10–11, Canada.

Hawthorn, D. (2006) Enhancing the contribution of older people to interface design. Gerontechnology, 5(1):4–14.

Ho, G., Wheatley, D., Scialfa, C.T. (2005) Age differences in trust and reliance of a medication management system. Interacting with Computers, 17:690–710.

Hopkins, H. (2007) Hitwise Intelligence. Source: http://weblogs.hitwise.com/heather-hopkins/2007/05/54_increase_put_silver_surfers.html, accessed 18 May 2007.

Intille, S.S. (2004) A new research challenge: persuasive technology to motivate healthy aging. IEEE Transactions on Information Technology in Biomedicine, 8(3):235–237.

Jacko, J., Emery, V.K., Edwards, P.J., Ashok, M., Barnard, L., Kongnakorn, T., Moloney, K.P., Sainfort, F. (July–August 2004) Effects of multimodal feedback on older adults' task performance given varying levels of computer experience. Behaviour & Information Technology, 23(4):247–264.

Jeffrey, S. (2003) Over 60s Reach for the Mouse, July 8 2003, www.guardian.co.uk, accessed on 18 October 2006.

Keates, S., Clarkson, P.J. (2003) The Design of Kiosks for Providing Access to E-Information for Older Adults, www.eng.cam.ac.uk, accessed 18 October 2006.

Lines, L., Hone, K. (2004) Eliciting user requirements with older adults: Lessons from the design of an interactive domestic alarm system. Universal Access in the Information Society, 3:141–148.

May, A., Ross, T., Osman, Z. (2005) The design of next generation in-vehicle navigation systems for the older driver. Interacting with Computers, 17:643–659.

Mynatt, E., Melenhorst, A., Fisk, A., Rogers, W. (2004) Aware technologies for ageing in place: Understanding user needs and attitudes. IEEE Pervasive Computing, 3(2):36–41.

McKenna, S.J., Marquis-Faulkes, F., Newell, A.F., Gregor, P. (2006) Requirements gathering using drama for computer vision-based monitoring in supportive home environments. Technology and Disability, 17(4):227–236.

Newell, A.F., Gregor, P. (2000). User sensitive inclusive design, in search of a new paradigm. Proceedings on the 2000 Conference on Universal Usability, pp. 39–44, November 16–17, 2000 (J. Scholtz, J. Thomas, eds.).

Norman, D.A. (1992) The Psychology of Everyday Things. Basic Books, New York.

Onn, I.L.Y., Jin, P.C.W. (1999) Assessment of the Elderly Patient. The Singapore Family Physician, 25(2), 1999. Available at: http://www.cfps.org.sg/sfp/25/252/articles/e252008.html, accessed 11 July 2006.

Perry, M., Dowdall, A., Lines, L., Hone, K. (2004) Multimodal and ubiquitous computing systems: Supporting independent-living older users. IEEE Transactions on Information Technology in Biomedicine, 8(3):258–270.

World Health Organisation. (2005) Preventing Chronic Diseases – A Vital Investment. Available at: http://www.who.int/chp/chronic_disease_report/contents/en/index.html. Accessed 2 January 2010.

Savitch, N., Zaphiris, P. (2005) An investigation into the accessibility of web-based information for people with dementia. Eleventh International Conference on Human-Computer Interaction, Las Vegas, July 2005.

Schneiderman, B. (1996) Designing the User Interface: Strategies for Effective Human-Computer Interaction. Addison-Wesley Publishing Company, Reading, Massachusetts..

Stalker, K., Gilliard, J., Downs, M.G. (1999) Eliciting user perspectives on what works. International Journal of Geriatric Psychiatry, 14:120–134.

Stott, M. (1981) *Ageing for Beginners*. Oxford, Blackwell.

Stuart-Hamilton, I. (1994) The Psychology of Ageing: An Introduction, 2nd edn. Kingsley, London.

van Horen, F., Jansen, C., Noordman, L., Maes, A. (2005) Manuals for the elderly: Text characteristics that help or hinder older users. IEEE International Professional Communication Conference Proceedings, Santa Fe, New Mexico.

Weiser, M. (September 1991) The computer for the 21st century. Scientific American, 265(3): 94–104.

Wright, P., Bartram, C., Rogers, N., Emslie, H., Evans, J., Wilson, B., Belt, S. (2000) Text entry on handheld computers by older users. Ergonomics, 43(6):702–716.

Zajicek, M. (2001) Interface Design for Older Adults. WUAUC'01, May 22–25, p. 60.

Zajicek, M., Brewster, S. (June 2004) Design principles to support older adults. Universal Access in the Information Society, 3(2):111–113.

Part IV
Evaluation and Assessment of Cognitive Prosthetics

Chapter 12
Practical Issues when Planning for Field Trials

Susanne Andersson and Anna-Lena Andersson

Abstract This chapter is written from a test site leader perspective and describes the role of planning and timing of field trials when testing technical solutions, which could enable people with dementia to live a more independent life. The chapter is based on experiences from setting up the first and second field trials in the three test sites of the COGKNOW project. The intention is to point out some key issues that are important in preparation and planning of a field trial. The chapter addresses issues in the preparatory, the actual and the post-test phase of the field trial in order to help achieve a high level of success both from a general perspective and with a special focus on people with dementia.

12.1 Introduction

The COGKNOW project iterates over three cycles of development, and each cycle comprises identification of user need, translated into requirements, which is implemented into a solution. The technical solution is tested in a field trial, before the solution is evaluated from various perspectives. In this chapter, the focus is the field trials, and specifically on the experiences of the three sites in the project – Amsterdam, Belfast and Luleå – as the first two of three field trials take place. The chapter explores the issues before, during and after each of the first two field trials, and indicates how success can be achieved in these scenarios.

S. Andersson (✉)
Division of Medical Specialities, Norrbotten County Council, Luleå, Sweden
e-mail: susanne.b.andersson@nll.se

M.D. Mulvenna, C.D. Nugent (eds.), *Supporting People with Dementia Using Pervasive Health Technologies*, Advanced Information and Knowledge Processing, DOI 10.1007/978-1-84882-551-2_12, © Springer-Verlag London Limited 2010

12.2 Preparatory Phase

Prior to a field trial several preparatory activities have to be conducted. For this reason preparation has to start early enough to ensure that there is time to carry out all of these activities. During this phase the base for the field trial is set. Continuous dialogue and cooperation between clinicians, researchers, technical developers and the participants/people with dementia and their relatives is necessary in order to reach a consensus of what functions to test and what to achieve during the trial. An overall responsible person, a field trial leader, ensures that there is a structure and planning for all the actions needed in order to set up and conduct each field trial.

The recruitment of users is done early, generally a couple of months before the planned starting date of each field trial, via networks for the target group, meeting centres and clinical departments. To succeed in recruitment it is important to explain the aim, goals and procedures involved in the field trials. It is also important to reassure the participants that their anonymity will be protected by the use of subject numbers.

All persons involved should have an agreed and committed Master Plan regarding each field trial with the following suggested content:

- The overall aim with the trial;
- Which functions to be tested during the trial;
- Starting point of the trial;
- Duration of the trial;
- Number of participants and inclusion criteria;
- Milestones – release dates of functions, purchase and delivery of equipment, etc.;
- Deadline of when pre-trial interviews and other pre-trial info is needed; and
- Named responsible persons for the different tasks "connected" to the field trial.

Before the field trial starts, it is essential that the different functionalities to be used during the trial are tested in a laboratory environment by the partners responsible for the technology. This is done to confirm that the hardware and software components of the devices and their services are stable, and that the functionalities requested are working in a satisfactory way – in other words to check that the technical equipment is operational. During the preparatory phase it is important that the equipment needed in the field trial is delivered from the technical partners to the trial site/s well in advance of trial start up. This makes it possible for the staff on each trial site to test the functionalities and check the stability of the system on site and also gives the people involved a chance to learn how the system works. On site testing is preferably led by the technician, the site technical partner, in close cooperation with the overall responsible site leader. Configuration and personalisation of the system are done by technical and clinical staff before the field trial starts.

Standardised methods of data collection for the field trial are constructed in the preparatory phase. Approximately 1 month before the starting date, a pre-trial interview/pre-trial visit is conducted, where information essential for a successful outcome is collected. A checklist is used to ensure that all important aspects will be covered. During the visit information regarding personalisation of the system is gathered. Personalisation is done in close cooperation with the users to meet their requests and needs. Pictures, phone numbers, type of reminders, layout of the screen are all examples of this. It is also important to check that the users still fulfil the inclusion criteria. If they meet the criteria they are asked to sign an informed consent. At this time appointments are made with each user for their individual starting date and length of the trial. It is also important to assess the home environment in preparation for the installation procedures.

Different kinds of user manuals are needed both prior to and during the field trial. For the technical partners an installation and user manual is necessary for setup and configuration. The clinical staff need a manual to guide them through the use of the system. The users/carers need a user manual which simply describes the functions of the system and helps them in their daily use.

Before the actual field trial the users are offered pre-test training. In the training sessions the latest functionality of the system is explained. The format of the trial is explained in detail. The pre-training sessions can either be given on an individual basis in the users homes or in a group session in a public location, for example, a meeting centre. Both options should involve a hands-on operation of the system assisted by clinical and technical staff in order to get familiar with the system. It is important at this stage, to reassure all participants that they will have access to a help desk throughout the trial. Thorough preparation in the preparatory phase is the key to success.

12.3 Actual Trial Phase

During the field trial the technical partner has a responsibility for the smooth operation of the equipment.

Before the field trial starts the equipment is installed in the user's home. Installation is facilitated by information collected during the pre-trial phase. Then a full demonstration is carried out by the clinical staff/researcher with support from the technical partner. The information and instructions given should preferably be personalised to each user and carer. The user manual is left in the home so that the users have access to support. In conjunction with the installation, tests and observations of the person with dementia will be made by the researcher.

During the field trial period it is important to set up a helpdesk. The function of the helpdesk is crucial to achieve a successful field trial. At each site the nominated technical partner is responsible for solving technical problems. They are the contact point for the users and the clinicians/researchers. During the field trial, it is essential to solve all problems promptly to facilitate the smooth running of the trial. This means that the technical partners need to be available at all times. The users and carers are given a direct telephone number and an e-mail address to the helpdesk in order to report problems as they occur.

Automatic logging of usage of the system is done during the field trial in order to get an overview of how the system is used. This is done by digital in situ measurements. In order to identify difficulties and problems during the field trial a bottle neck list, a kind of diary, will be filled in by the users, or if needed, by the clinicians/researchers. This is helpful in order to collect information about potential improvement issues or actual problems of any kind in the system from the user perspective. In this event the technical partners can identify the urgency of a problem, find the solution and make future improvements. The bottle neck list should identify areas for improvement.

Regular telephone calls or follow-up visits during the field trial are essential to monitor the participants' use of the system and to see how everything is going generally. This is necessary in order to identify any difficulties not reported to the help desk. In practice, some users may require more support than others in using the system.

At the end of the trial the initial tests and observations are repeated by the researchers.

12.4 Post-test Procedure

A formal end point is agreed between all persons involved. After the field trial has ended the technical partner has the important role of uninstalling the system. It is essential for all staff to respect the participant's home and ensure that it is left as it was prior to installation. It is also important to maintain contact after the field trial ends so that any remaining issues can be addressed. When the result of the overall field trial is analysed the participants will receive feedback. This can be done individually or in a workshop.

12.5 Conclusions

To have a successful outcome of the field trial we would like to point out that it is important that agreements about deadlines and appointments are respected, since changes affect all persons involved including the person with dementia and their carers. If there are multiple changes of appointments there is a risk that the participants will become de-motivated and/or withdraw consent. It is also essential that all persons involved, technical, clinical and test persons, have the same perspective and understanding about the overall goal with the project and also what to achieve and what is expected in every single field trial. In all projects involving technology and test persons there will most likely be ups and downs. Especially in the beginning of the project, in the first field trial loop difficulties with the technology might occur more frequently since the development just started. As time passes and the technology becomes more mature and developed, the system stability increases and the outcome of the field trials will result in a higher success rate.

Conducting field trials in the homes of the people with dementia also might influence the trial in a way since the trial is done on the terms of the person with dementia. The staff have to remember that they are guests in their house. This means that the home needs to be seen as a *home* and not as a test laboratory. This is also an ethical view that gives empowerment to the person with dementia and their relatives.

The benefit from working with iterative field trials is that it is a learning process. From each field trial you bring the best of it into the following field trial and improves the quality and result each time.

Chapter 13
Evaluation of Cognitive Prosthetics

Stefan Sävenstedt, Franka Meiland, Rose-Marie Dröes, and Ferial Moelaert

Abstract An important aspect when developing assistive technical services for persons with dementia is the assessment of usability and usefulness from the perspective of the user. The COGKNOW project aims at developing an assistive device for persons with mild dementia and the evaluation of the first pilot device was based on a multiple case study design using mainly a qualitative approach in data collection. The design of the evaluation used a mix method approach using semi-structured interviews, combining structured and open questions, and semi-structured observations. Persons with dementia provide special challenges in assessing usefulness and user friendliness due to their cognitive impairments. The experiences from the first test of the COGKNOW device showed that the use of a mix method approach provides a comprehensive understanding of the usefulness and user friendliness that overcome some of the challenges.

13.1 Introduction

The assessment of to what extent assistive technology can support persons with dementia in facilitating their daily life activities and support experiences that promote well-being and independence is an area of vital concern that has been limitedly explored (Margot-Cattin and Nygård 2006). An important aspect when developing such technical devices is the assessment of usability and usefulness from the perspective of the person with dementia. A major challenge in such assessment is the methodology aspects on how to best understand, measure and interpret their experiences.

Many studies aiming at exploring the experiences and lifeworld of persons with dementia have used a qualitative approach, using interviews or systematic observations as a mean to gather information. Qualitative interviewing and analysis

S. Sävenstedt (✉)
Centre for Distance-Spanning Healthcare, Luleå University of Technology, Luleå, Sweden
e-mail: stefan.savenstedt@ltu.se

techniques provide an opportunity to obtain a detailed, flexible in-depth understanding of individuals' beliefs and perceptions relating to a particular issue (Lloyd et al. 2006; Patton 2002). At the same time there is an identifiable and consistent pattern in interview research of recruiting only those individuals with the likely ability to articulate their views. In interviewing the persons with dementia, mainly persons with mild to moderate and severe dementia, who do not have aphasia, will be able to participate. Because of this, interview research conducted with persons who have dementia remains significantly limited compared to research involving the general population (Lloyd et al. 2006). Reviews of interview studies conducted with persons with dementia confirm, despite the challenges of problems of expression, that it is possible to study their experiences in a way that is meaningful using adapted interview strategies (Moore and Hollett 2003).

One means of overcoming the difficulties in attempting to interview individuals with expressive language problems have been to seek the views of carers or proxy respondents instead. However, the experiences are that such an approach is likely to provide more information about the experiences and subjectivity of the carers or proxies than about the individual person with dementia (Kitwood 1997). On the other hand it has been argued by researchers that the observations of carers can be regarded as more valid information than the expressed information of persons with communication and cognitive impairments (Hubbard et al. 2003).

Observations of the activities of the person with dementia are another indirect way of understanding how the person with dementia experiences aspects such as usefulness and user friendliness of assistive devices. Observation studies of persons with dementia are most common with persons in moderate to severe stages of the disease. However, observations used as complement to simultaneous open interviews can provide advantages when the informants are in a mild or moderate stage of dementia. An example of this approach was used in an evaluation study of the use of assistive technology to support safety among persons with dementia in a group dwelling. The study showed that the use of an ethnographic approach, involving both spontaneous open interviews in combination with participant observations provided reach and relevant data for the evaluation (Nygård 2006).

There are many examples of research carried out with persons who have dementia using structured or semi-structured questionnaires and validated interview instruments in order to assess subjective experiences such as quality of life and sense of autonomy. Important experience when using structured questionnaires in interviews with persons who have a mild or moderate dementia is that, in order to maintain attention, it should be brief. Special techniques such as presenting the questions and response scales both orally and visually can help the person to attend to questions and choose the right alternative (Trigg et al. 2007). One main advantage of using structured questionnaires and validated interview instruments is the possibility of comparing results with other research. There are also examples of researchers who have used a combination of validated instruments, structured questionnaires and logged data in the evaluation of the use of technical devices by persons with dementia (Shoval et al. 2008; van der Roest et al. 2008). A key issue in assessments of aspects of daily living among persons with dementia using different scales is the sensitivity of the scales. Contexts vary and one problem of sensitivity is that the process of incorporating what follows from changes in the society, as the use of technological equipments, is slow in many scales (Nygård and Winblad 2006).

Several authors have argued that the use of mixed methods and a triangulation of different data collection methods provide a more accurate and complete account than any single method could on its own (Maxwell 1996; Patton 2002). On the other hand there are also problems linked to the use of mixed methods where the internal consistency and logic of each research approach can create difficulties. For example, a qualitative phenomenological approach used to understand the meaning the person with dementia gives to technical devices can from a philosophical view be difficult to combine with a quantitative approach using experimental design. However, using a practical approach where the research question is in focus and not epistemological and philosophical arguments, problems can be overcome with adaptability and creativity in designing studies (Patton 2002).

In this chapter we describe how the evaluation of usefulness and user friendliness of the first COGKNOW pilot device was conducted together with experiences drawn from the evaluation. Reflections and conclusions for future field studies are also presented.

13.2 Evaluation Design

The design of the human factor analysis, of the one out of three field tests of the COGKNOW device, was based on a multiple case study design using mainly a qualitative approach in data collection. It was aiming at developing theoretical aspects on usefulness and user friendliness (Yin 1994). The design of the evaluation focused on collecting data from three perspectives, the person with dementia, their family member or carer and the researcher. Data were collected both through semi-structured interviews, combining structured and open questions and through semi-structured observations. In addition "in situ" measurements in the form of logged data about the use of devices during the test were collected.

13.2.1 Settings

The field study was carried out in the participants' homes at three test sites; one in Amsterdam in The Netherlands, a second in Belfast in Northern Ireland and a third in Luleå, Sweden.

13.2.2 Procedures

Common guidelines regarding the inclusion criteria and methods of data collection were agreed upon by all test sites, allowing for comparison of data between sites.

All participating persons with dementia were, together with the family members/carers, checked against the inclusions criteria for participants during the spring of 2007. A consent agreement was signed by all participants. Context data to describe similarities and differences between the participants were also collected prior to the test.

The evaluation activities at each test site were managed quite independently by local research teams, but several coordination meetings and joint planning sessions were conducted in order to secure a common approach. The descriptive and analytic results from each test site were first analysed separately by the local teams and thereafter put together as common result for the human factor analysis of all three test sites.

In Northern Ireland and in The Netherlands the installation, test interviewing and de-installation of the equipment were conducted on the same day, approximately 4–5 h in total. In Sweden the equipment was installed 1 day in advance before testing, with the exception of one case where the installation was made 6 days prior to testing. In The Netherlands and in Northern Ireland the field-test interviewing of both the person with dementia and the family member/carer was completed within approximately 2 h, whereas in Sweden prolonged interviewing sessions were conducted, the researchers spending on average 4–5 h together with the informants. The Swedish approach gave probably the opportunity to a firmer acquaintance with the users and with the prototype prior to testing. In Northern Ireland and in The Netherlands the user instructions were provided prior to testing.

The semi-structured interview questionnaire used in the field test was developed through a rigorous process, starting with formulating detailed research questions. The research questions covered both general aspects and aspects of usefulness and user friendliness in the four main areas of daily living that the COGKNOW device was designed to assist. The four areas were social communication, support of memory, safety and daily activities. The questionnaire had a design with several detailed questions with fixed response alternatives, combined with open questions in all areas. The evaluation used the same questionnaire for both the person with dementia and the family member/carer.

The field-test interviews concentrated on the users' interactions with the hardware, touch screen, mobile device and sensors and the four main functionalities of the COGKNOW device. A pre-configured prototype, fixed reminders, fixed photographs for the calling system, fixed music facilities and a standard warning sensor for open doors were applied during testing. The persons with dementia performed prescribed tasks to allow researchers to observe the interaction with the device.

General questions about the size, shape and weight of the equipment were administrated to the participants, as well as about their charging of the mobile device. The screen size, readability of text, audibility of the alarms and handling of bottoms were checked in a structured manner guided by a fixed approach. Open questions about the specific usefulness of the functions installed, and about the user friendliness of these functionalities as seen from the user's point of views, were administrated to all informants. In addition there were also some questions regarding the easiness of learning how to use the device asked.

Semi-structured observations were conducted by the researchers during the test on the users handling of the COGKNOW device, covering aspects of four prioritised functionality areas.

There was a slight difference of the timing of the test between the three test sites, allowing slight adjustment and adaptations of the technical performance of the COGKNOW device. Even if the adjustments carried out were minor, the conditions and the technical performance of the device were not exactly the same at all three test sites.

13.2.3 Analysis

For the analysis, SPSS data files covering structured questions and a code scheme for the qualitative content analyses of open questions were agreed upon between the sites. Each site performed the analyses of its own data, but several coordination meetings and joint planning sessions were conducted in order to secure a common approach. The results of the three test sites were compared and summarised resulting in a common integrated human factor analysis of all three test sites.

13.2.4 Participants

Selection of the dyad of a person with dementia and a family member/carer for the test was based on the inclusion criteria of the person with dementia having a diagnosis of dementia of the Alzheimer type, as described in the DSM-IV-TR. In addition they should be assessed through the standardised Brief Cognitive Rating Scale (Reisberg 1983) as suffering from mild dementia, described in the Global Deterioration Scale as level 3, 4 or 5. The participants should be willing and able to participate actively in the different evaluation activities. The close person or informal carer should be regularly in contact with or care for the person with dementia. An overview of participants in the field test is provided in Table 13.1.

Table 13.1 Characteristics of participants in field test #1

Participants	Amsterdam	Belfast	Luleå
Persons with dementia	$N = 5$	$N = 6$	$N = 5$
Mean age (years)	64.7 (range 56–78)	72.7 (range 65–86)	67.8 (range 60–77)
Gender	3 female	5 female	3 female
	2 male	1 male	2 male
Civil status	4 married	3 married	5 married
	1 divorced	2 widowed	
		1 single	
Family members/carers	$N = 5$	$N = 6$	$N = 5$
Mean age (years)	59.2 (range 49–78)	53.0 (range 40–72)	61.4 (range 23–78)
Gender	3 female	3 female	2 female
	2 male	3 male	3 male
Relation to patient	4 spouses	3 spouses	4 spouses
	1 daughter	2 children	1 son
		1 cousin	

13.3 Experiences from the Evaluation

The design of the evaluation of the usefulness and user friendliness of the first COGKNOW prototype device raised several issues on both collecting data and performing the analysis.

13.3.1 Interviewing the Person with Dementia

For the person with dementia it was obvious that in order to keep their attention to the questions and the fixed responses of the detailed questions, the questions had to be posed at the same time as a function of the device was used. The specific function had to be valued while performing the action. An example was the questions on the picture-dialling function. When posing the question "How do you judge the picture-dialling function?" with the fixed responses, helpful, appropriate and not very helpful, it was very essential to go through the different steps of the function at the same time.

A specific problem in the evaluation was when a technical problem with performance of the COGKNOW prototype occurred. An example was when the call-up function of the picture dialling was not working properly or when the sound of the receiver was badly adjusted, the attention of the person with dementia was distracted. The abstract thinking of valuing a function in the way as it was intended to work while not performing well seemed very difficult to comprehend. A conclusion was that the function or aspect of the function could only be valued if it was fully working and technical problems made the participants lose attention.

Open questions like "How do you judge the picture-dialling service?" gave valuable additional information. Through these types of questions it was possible for the person with dementia to formulate their impression in their own words. A challenge was to stimulate them to narrate by using follow-up questions on function, interaction and experiences of usefulness and user friendliness. These were questions like "What do you think about using these pictures when making a call?" "Will these pictures facilitate you making calls?" and "How do you think about this way of making calls compared to the usual way?" An important experience with the open questions posed to the person with dementia was, in the same way as the structured questions, that they had to be posed in the immediate connection to the use of the function on the device. More abstract open questions like "Do you have suggestions to improve the picture-dialling function?" were more difficult to the answerer and relate to for most of the persons with dementia. Some of the participants could give valuable suggestions when more concrete follow-up questions like "Should the pictures look this way or what do you think about the steps you have to make when making a call?"

13.3.2 Interviewing the Family Member/Carer

The family member/carer answered a semi-structured questionnaire that looked almost the same as the one that was used in the interview with the person with dementia. Looking at similarities and differences between the answers of the family member/carer and the persons with dementia it was obvious that there were more similarities than differences and few contradictive answers between the two perspectives. One area where sometimes there were different opinions between the person with dementia and the family member was in the case of assessing usefulness in relation to needs. There were several examples where the person with dementia had the opinion that they were not in need of a function while the family member/carer could see the usefulness.

Another difference was that the family member/carer could provide additional information on the more abstract questions. Questions like how to develop the device further, the possibility of the person with dementia to learn how to use the device and general questions on the usability of a function or general aspects of the device. In the open questions the family member/carer could provide information on how the person with dementia used to behave in a similar situation and compare that experience with the performance of the device. An example on additional information on usability was the suggestion by some family members to relate the picture-dialling function to the lack of ability of some of the persons with dementia to remember important phone numbers and to initiate social phone calls. On the aspect of user friendliness the family member/carer could as an example provide additional information related to their experience on the ability of the person with dementia to learn how to use new technical devices and their ability to read text and interpret symbols.

13.3.3 Observations

The interaction of the person with dementia and the COGKNOW device was also observed by the researchers during the test. The observations had an open structure following an observation scheme outlining important areas to be observed. It was designed to facilitate comparisons between the users at the three test sites and covered besides contextual information, information on the performance of the device and also interaction aspects of the four main areas of daily activities that the device was designed to assist with.

The observations provided valuable information on how the person with dementia interacted with the different functions of the device together with information about spontaneous reaction when interacting. As an example, it was possible to observe if the person with dementia could identify the right icon for the function he was willing to initiate as the icon for making telephone calls. If they could remember to perform the different steps of conducting a phone call and at what situations they had problems of understanding what to do. It was also possible to observe how they responded to preset reminders on making a certain call and if they could take action, confirm the reminder and in a next step performed the action of calling.

13.3.4 In Situ Measurements

Some of the research questions are partly approached by "in situ" measurements which measure phenomena through logged traffic data such as frequency and timing of specific use of different function areas. The "in situ" measurement was performed through specially developed software SeniorXensor (Mulder et al. 2005) that registered the use of the mobile device. As an example the software could log when the mobile was used, which function of the device was used and to whom the person with dementia made calls.

13.3.5 Experiences of the Analysis Process

The analyses of the different data were conducted with a design for mix methods where quantitative data were validated with qualitative data (Creswell et al. 2007). Based on specific research questions, quantitative and qualitative data were first analysed separately. Thereafter the quantitative and qualitative data from different perspectives were compared and a final interpretation was carried out.

The mix method analysis approach allowed us to add interesting and more embellished information with nuances to the structural data from the person with dementia and the family member/carer. Observations by the researchers provided additional and valuable information on how the person with dementia performed when using the different functions of the COGKNOW devices. As an example, most of the persons with dementia confirmed in the structural data that it was easy to use and understand the picture directory of the communication function. They could also give more elaborative comments in the open questions that gave additional information on what aspects of the function that was more difficult to comprehend. The family members/carers supported this with their answers on the structural and open questions. The researcher could observe how the person with dementia carried out the different steps of the calling process. In the concluding integrated analysis we could confirm that all different data showed that the concept of picture dialling worked well. There were some problems with the different steps of the process that seemed to complicate the calling and needed to be simplified.

At this first round of tests of the COGKNOW devices we were not able to include the logged "in situ" measurements since it was connected to the mobile device that had a low technical performance at this stage. We anticipate that this type of data will give valuable additional information in the evaluation of the devices in the second and third rounds of test when the devices will be tested during a longer time period.

13.4 Discussion

The COGKNOW project aims at being a user-centric project and one of the main challenges from the point of view of evaluation is to understand usability and user friendliness from the perspective of the person with dementia. The challenges of understanding their thinking and perceptions are well documented by many researchers (Kitwood 1997; Lloyd et al. 2006; Nygård 2006). The use of a mix method design in the first test of the COGKNOW prototype has according to our experiences proved to be valuable.

The mix method evaluation design for assessing usability and user friendliness of assistive technical services has it own challenges. Even though it is easy to accept that the use of mixed methods provides a more accurate and complete account than any single method could on its own (Maxwell 1996; Patton 2002), there are many researchers disputing the possibility of handling different research paradigms in the same evaluation process (Creswell and Plano Clark 2007). As in all research, the research problems should guide the design and it can be argued that mixed method research is more suited for some problems than others. The benefit of using a mixed method design for assessing the use of assistive technology by people with mild dementia has been confirmed by other researchers (Nygård 2006). Many researchers have also showed the possibility of handling different research paradigm in the same evaluation process (Creswell and Plano Clark 2007).

The use of a multiple case study design in the evaluation process of technical devices provided several benefits. The main benefit was that we could build our theoretical understanding of usability and user friendliness of the device for persons with dementia (cf. Yin 1994). A specific advantage of using a multiple case study design, with participants from three different countries, is that we achieved a variation among the participants in many variables, such as the way of living and previous experiences of technical devices. A variation that increased the trustworthiness of the results (Yin 1994; Patton 2002). A specific problem in evaluations of technical prototypes is that the number of devices is limited and does not allow tests with many participants. This is an additional argument for the benefit of using a case study design.

13.5 Conclusion

The experiences from the evaluation process in the first round of test of the COGKNOW device confirm the benefits of using a multiple case study design with a mixed method approach. A user-centric design process requires a good understanding of how the user perceives the usability and user friendliness of the different prototypes. Persons with dementia provide special challenges in this aspect due to their cognitive impairments. The use of mixed data collection methods as open and structural questions in interviews, together with interviews with family members/carers, and observations by researchers provide a comprehensive understanding that overcomes some of these challenges. In future tests of the device we believe that logged "in situ" measurements will provide valuable additional information that will improve the evaluation process.

References

Creswell, J.W., Plano Clark, V.L. (2007) Designing and Conducting Mixed Methods Research, Vol. 1. Thousand Oaks, Sage Publications.

Hubbard, G., Downs, M., Tester, S. (2003) Including older people with dementia in research: Challenges and strategies. Aging and Mental Health, 7:351–362.

Kitwood, T. (1997). Dementia reconsidered: The person comes first. Buckingham, U.K.: Open University Press.

Lloyd, V., Gatherer, A., Kalsy, S. (2006) Conducting qualitative interview research with people with expressive language difficulties. Qualitative Health Research, 16(10):1386–1404.

Margot-Cattin, I., Nygård, L. (2006) Access technology and dementia care: Influences on residents' everyday lives in a secure unit. Scandinavian Journal of Occupational Therapy, 13:113–124.

Maxwell, J.A. (1996) Qualitative Research Design: An Interactive Approach. Thousand Oaks, Sage publications.

Moore, T.F., Hollett, J. (2003) Giving voice to persons living with dementia: The researcher's opportunities and challenges. Nursing Science Quarterly, 16(2):163–167.

Mulder, I., ter Hofte, G.H., Kort, J. (2005) Socio Xensor: Measuring user behavior and user eXperience in conteXt with mobile device. Paper presented at the Measuring Behavior 2005, the 5th International Conference on Methods and Techniques in Behavioral Research, 30 August–2 September, 2005, Wageningen, The Netherlands.

Nygård, L. (2006) How can we get access to the experiences of people with dementia? Suggestions and reflections. Scandinavian Journal of Occupational Therapy, 13:101–112.

Nygård, L., Winblad, B. (2006) Measuring long term effects and changes in the daily activities of people with dementia. The Journal of Nutrition, Health and Aging, 10(2):137–138.

Patton, M. (2002) Qualitative Research & Evaluation Methods, 3rd edn. Sage Publications Inc., Thousands Oaks.

Shoval, N., Auslander, G.K., Freytag, T., Landau, R., Oswald, F., Seidl, U. et al. (2008) The use of advanced tracking technologies for the analysis of mobility in Alzheimer's disease and related cognitive diseases. BMC Geriatrics, 8:7.

Reisberg, B. (1983) The brief cognitive rating scale and global deterioration scale. In: T. Crook, S. Ferris, C. Bartus (eds.) Assets in Geriatric Psychopharmacology. Mark Powley Ass. Inc., New Canaan, CT, pp. 19–35.

Trigg, R., Skevington, S.M., Jones, R.W. (2007) How can we best assess the quality of life of people with dementia? The Bath Assessment of Subjective Quality of Life in Dementia (BASQID). Gerontologist, 47(6):789–797.

Van der Roest, H.G., Meiland, F.J.M., Jonker, C., Dröes, R.M. (2008). User evaluation of the DEMentia-specific Digital Interactive Social Chart (DEM-DISC). A Pilot study among informal carers on its impact, user friendliness and usefulness, Aging and Mental Health, (in press).

Yin, R.K. (1994) Case Study Research, 2nd edn., Vol. 5. Thousand Oaks, SAGE Publications.

Chapter 14
Measuring the Impact of Cognitive Prosthetics on the Daily Life of People with Dementia and Their Carers

Franka Meiland, Rose-Marie Dröes, and Stefan Sävenstedt

Abstract Assistive technologies to support persons with dementia and their carers are used increasingly often. However, little is known about the effectiveness of most assistive devices. Much technology is put on the market without having been properly tested with potential end-users. To increase the chance that an assistive device is well accepted and useful for the target group, it is important, especially in the case of disabled persons, to involve potential users in the development process and to evaluate the impact of using the device on them before implementing it in the daily care and support. When evaluating the impact, decisions have to be made regarding the selection of measuring instruments. Important considerations in the selection process are the underlying domains to be addressed by the assistive technology, the target group and the availability of standardized instruments with good psychometric properties. In this chapter the COGKNOW project is used as a case example to explain how the impact of cognitive prosthetics on the daily lives of people with dementia and their carers can be measured. In COGKNOW a cognitive prosthetic device is being developed to improve the quality of life and autonomy of persons with dementia and to help them to remember and remind, to have social contact, to perform daily activities and to enhance feelings of safety. For all these areas, potential measuring instruments are described. Besides (standardized) measuring instruments, other data collection methods are used as well, such as semi-structured interviews and observations, diaries and in situ measurement. Within the COGKNOW project a first uncontrolled small-scale impact measurement takes place during the development process of the assistive device. However, it is recommended to perform a larger randomized controlled study as soon as the final product is ready to evaluate the impact of the device on persons with dementia and carers before it is released on the market.

F. Meiland (✉)
Department of Psychiatry, Alzheimer Centre, VU University Medical Centre/GGZ Buitenamstel, Valeriusplein, Amsterdam, The Netherlands
e-mail: fj.meiland@vumc.nl

M.D. Mulvenna, C.D. Nugent (eds.), *Supporting People with Dementia Using Pervasive Health Technologies*, Advanced Information and Knowledge Processing, DOI 10.1007/978-1-84882-551-2_14, © Springer-Verlag London Limited 2010

14.1 Introduction

In recent years, assistive technologies are being used increasingly often to support people with dementia and their carers (ASTRID 2000; Nugent 2007). Some of these technologies were studied on their effectiveness in persons with dementia and their carers (Lauriks et al., 2007). However, most of these studies show methodologi-cal shortcomings, such as the use of very small groups, uncontrolled study designs, and the application of unstandardized measuring instruments. Results from a recent review suggest that there is a need for testing new ICT solutions in controlled studies in real-life situations, before implementing them in the care and support for persons with dementia (Lauriks et al., 2007). In designing this research, it has to be decided which outcome measures are appropriate to test the impact of the device in the daily life of the users. When implementing a device for persons with dementia living in the community, it can be expected that the device might have an impact not only on the persons with dementia but also on their informal carers. Sixty-five per cent of the persons with dementia are living in the community and are cared for by infor-mal carers like spouses or children, sometimes assisted by professional caregivers (Health Council 2002).

In this chapter we will describe our considerations on measuring the impact of a cognitive prosthetic device on the daily life of persons with dementia and their carers. We will use the European COGKNOW project as a case example and there-fore will first describe the aims of this project, the prosthetic device that is developed and the impact on daily life that is intended with the device to be developed. After that we will discuss the methods we selected in this project to measure the impact on the daily life of persons with dementia and their carers. Some of these methods were tried out in a previous phase of the project. We will evaluate these methods and give recommendations for measuring the impact in future field studies into the effect of assistive technology.

14.2 Aims of the COGKNOW Project and Potential Impact

The goal of the COGKNOW project is to develop a cognitive prosthetic device that will have an impact on the daily life of persons with dementia and their carers.[1] The device aims to enhance the quality of life and the (actual and perceived) autonomy of persons with dementia. The device that is developed is called the COGKNOW Day Navigator (CDN) and consists of a stationary component (touch screen), a mobile component and sensors. The CDN has several functionalities to support persons with dementia in four areas, namely remembering and reminding, social contact, daily activities and (feelings of) safety. These areas were chosen because needs assessment studies indicated that they were the most frequently experienced areas of unmet need for persons with dementia living in the community and their carers

---

[1] www.cogknow.eu

(van der Roest et al. 2007; Miranda and Orrell 2008). In the area of remembering and reminding the CDN reminds persons with dementia about the current day and time by an analogue clock on the touch screen and by pop-up reminders to perform activities or to remember appointments. An item locator service that is also available on the touch screen helps the person with dementia to find objects when lost, e.g. finding the mobile. In the area of social contact, persons with dementia are supported in making a phone call by means of a picture dialling service integrated in the touch screen as well. In the area of daily activities, persons with dementia are supported in using a music player and radio function by means of simple on/off buttons on the touch screen of the CDN persons with dementia can also receive video assistance when performing some daily activities, such as making a cup of tea or using the washing machine. And, finally, in the area of safety there is a help function that allows persons with dementia to easily make phone contact with an informal carer, and sensor-based safety warnings that pop-up in case of unsafe situations, for instance when a door is left open.

We can envision that using the CDN will enhance the quality of life of persons with dementia, for instance, by the experienced support in remembering appointments, by engaging in joyful activities such as listening to music and by feeling more secure because of the safety warnings one receives in case of potential danger. Also, the actual and perceived autonomy may be influenced by using the CDN: persons with dementia might become better in control of the activities they planned or need to perform, because of the calendar function and the support in day and time orientation. They might be enabled again to get in phone contact with their social network, because of the easy to operate picture dialling telephone.

14.3 Selection of Measuring Instruments to Evaluate the Impact of the CDN

In this section we will outline our considerations on the operationalization of the concepts of quality of life and autonomy and on the impact of the CDN on each specific functional area that is supported with the CDN. We will describe which measuring instruments we selected and why.

Besides the impact measures, it is certainly also important to evaluate whether the device is user-friendly and useful for persons with dementia and carers. This topic was already described elsewhere in the book so will not be discussed further here.

14.3.1 General Considerations When Selecting Impact Measures

When choosing impact measures for evaluating an intervention, several notions have to be considered:

• What underlying domains are addressed by a given intervention? (Moniz-Cook et al. 2008).

- At which target group is the intervention aimed? Can the target group be interviewed using questionnaires and/or open interviews; are observation measures preferred or should informal carers or other (professionals) provide information on the persons with dementia (so-called proxy measures).
- Are standardized instruments with good psychometric properties available for measuring the impact on the selected domains and target group? For instance, the reliability, validity and responsiveness to change of measuring instruments will have to be considered.

To make a comparison possible of the results of different psychosocial interventions, it is advised to use consensus instruments for the different domains (Moniz-Cook et al., 2008). Based on an iterative collaborative, evidence-based method, the INTERDEM[2] group recently published a comprehensive list of best outcome measures for European psychosocial interventions. Within COGKNOW we made use of this list in the selection of measuring instruments.

14.3.2 Considerations and Selection of Instruments in the COGKNOW Project

14.3.2.1 General Considerations in the COGKNOW Project

In the COGKNOW project, three iterative cycles are scheduled in 3 years time, in which different prototypes are evaluated with potential end-users and their carers in three countries (The Netherlands, Northern Ireland and Sweden). In the first two cycles, the evaluation focused on user-friendliness and usefulness of the prototype. In the third and last cycle, the evaluation mainly aims at studying the impact on the daily life of persons with dementia and their carers. This impact measurement pilot takes place during the development process of the CDN and it aims to explore the impact of the third prototype. Because the CDN is still a prototype, and not a stable end product, it is in this phase of the study not opportune to do a large randomized controlled study. At three test sites (in Amsterdam, Belfast and Luleå), we therefore will perform a small-scale one-group evaluation study with a total of 12 persons with mild dementia living in the community and their carers. Persons with dementia who are having severe aphasia will be excluded from the study, thus allowing all participants to be interviewed. In COGKNOW, we will use several evaluation methods: standardized measuring instruments if comparison with other studies is considered relevant; semi-structured interviews and diaries for detailed evaluation of the prototype and if no standardized measuring instruments are available and logging methods to assess the actual use of services of the CDN during the test period.

---

[2]European organization on early detection and timely psychosocial INTERventions in DEMentia.

14.3.2.2 Primary General Impact Measures

The main goal of the CDN is to enhance the quality of life and autonomy of persons with dementia. Quality of life is a generally applied and accepted outcome measure in psychogeriatric research since almost two decades (Lawton 1991; Rabins and Kasper 1997; Dröes et al. 1998; Brod et al., 1999; Logsdon et al., 1999; Ettema et al., 2005; Schölzel-Dorenbos 2007). Quality of life is a multidimensional concept, and opinions differ regarding which domains are considered important for one's quality of life. There are, for instance, differences between people with dementia, their professional caregivers and in literature what domains are regarded as relevant (Dröes et al., 2006). Since quality of life is a subjective construct, self-ratings are preferred above proxy measures. In Europe there is consensus that the quality of life in Alzheimer's Disease Scale (QoL-AD) (Logsdon et al., 1999) is the measure of choice (Moniz-Cook et al., 2008). Reasons for this are that it is a short questionnaire, it has demonstrated sensitivity to psychosocial intervention (Spector et al., 2003) and it is used internationally. The questionnaire consists of 13 questions on different aspects of life, such as physical health, mood, family and doing things for fun. Persons with dementia rate these 13 aspects as poor, fair, good or excellent. In the family version of the Qol-AD, the carers judge these aspects for the persons with dementia. Though it is not to be expected that all QoL-AD domains will be influenced by using the CDN, we prefer to use the full instrument. When using the full instrument we will be able to describe the study population's quality of life and to compare it with the quality of life of participants in other intervention studies. One domain that persons with dementia consider very important for their quality of life, and that might also be influenced by using the CDN, is "self-esteem". Because this domain is not addressed by the QoL-AD scale, a subscale of the Dementia Quality of Life instrument (D-QoL, Brod et al., 1999) might be added to assess self-esteem. However, this aspect could be evaluated in a semi-structured interview too. A safe environment is another aspect of quality of life that is considered important by persons with dementia and professional carers. As the CDN aims to enhance the feelings of safety, and this aspect is not included in the present measuring instruments on quality of life in dementia, we will include this subject in the semi-structured interview that we will compose specifically for COGKNOW.

As for the assessment of experienced autonomy no suitable instrument was available, we decided to compose a questionnaire for this ourselves. This so-called Experienced Autonomy questionnaire (Meiland and Dröes 2006) contains seven items from the Mastery Scale (Pearlin and Schooler 1978) and five items that we adapted from the WHOQOL100 (WHO 2002). The thus composed Experienced Autonomy list (see Appendix 1) consists of 12 statements, such as "I have little control over the things that happen to me", "I often feel helpless in dealing with the problems of life", "I feel I have difficulty performing everyday activities" and "I feel able to make decisions". These statements are read aloud to the persons with dementia and they are asked to indicate on a response card to what degree they agree with the statement on a five-point scale (from totally agree to totally disagree). We have tested this instrument in the first cycle of the COGKNOW project. People with dementia were able to respond, and responses showed good variation. However, the psychometric properties of the instrument are not known yet.

Besides experienced autonomy, also the actual autonomy may be influenced by using the CDN. This might be seen in, for instance, a decrease in the need of assistance. An Activity of Daily Living scale may be used to assess this potential impact (see Section 14.3.2.3, daily activities). Also, the actual performance of activities, such as making phone calls, may be logged.

As the CDN aims to fulfil some of the needs of people with dementia, the number of unmet needs is expected to decrease when using the CDN. Therefore, unmet needs are an outcome measure in this study as well. The unmet needs will be inventoried with the Camberwell Assessment of Need for the Elderly (CANE, Reynolds et al., 2000; translated into Dutch by Dröes et al. (2004)). The CANE assesses needs of elderly people on 24 domains of daily living and measures whether these needs are met or unmet. The instrument also contains two items directed particularly at the needs of informal carers. The CANE can record judgments on needs from the viewpoint of the elderly person, of the informal carer, of a professional and of an external assessor. The English and the Dutch version have good psychometric properties (Reynolds et al., 2000; van der Roest et al., 2008).

14.3.2.3 Impact Measures for the Four Areas of Support

Regarding the impact of support for *remembering and reminding*, we will assess with the CANE if people with dementia experience less problems in the area of memory. Also, people with dementia may be better oriented in time because they use the day and time indication on the CDN. This will be assessed by using single items of the Mini Mental State Examination (MMSE, Folstein et al., 1975; see also Section 14.3.2.5).

In the area of support in social contact, the number and quality of social contacts may improve because of the use of the picture dialling phone. This impact can be measured with one item of the QoL-AD (Logsdon et al., 1999) on interpersonal relations and with two items of the CANE (Reynolds et al., 2000) on company and intimate relationships.

In the area of support in daily activities, the activity assistance service aims to help people in their daily activities. The potential impact of this service may be assessed with an instrument on (instrumental) activities of daily living, of which many instruments are available. An instrument especially developed for people with dementia is the Interview for Deterioration in Daily living activities in Dementia (IDDD) which assesses the initiative to and the actual performance of self-care and more complex activities. This instrument has good psychometric properties ($\alpha=0.94$, Teunisse and Derix 1991).

In the area of enhancing feelings of safety, people with dementia may feel less anxious. A measuring instrument on anxiety that has been used in persons with dementia is the Rating Anxiety in Dementia (RAID; Shankar et al., 1999); however, until now this instrument lacks evidence of sensitivity to change (Moniz-Cook et al., 2008).

For each of the four areas, we will add a question in the semi-structured interview to assess whether and how the CDN helps persons with dementia to fulfil their needs.

14.3.2.4 Secondary Impact Measures

The use of the CDN may also influence other aspects of functioning. For instance, it may influence how persons with dementia cope with the consequences of their illness. A questionnaire that previously has been used (amongst others) with persons with dementia is the Jalowiec Coping Scale (JCS), an instrument that assesses the use and effectiveness of 60 cognitive and behavioural coping strategies (α-scores vary from 0.64 to 0.97) (Dröes 1996; Dröes et al., 2006). Another questionnaire on coping is the Dementia Coping questionnaire, an instrument that was developed specifically for the group of people with early stage dementia (Reinersmann et al., 2006; see Appendix 2). The psychometric properties of this questionnaire are yet unknown.

When persons with dementia benefit from using the CDN, this may also have a positive impact on the quality of life and experienced burden of their carers. Persons with dementia may function more independently and will be less demanding towards the carers, e.g. by asking less questions to the carer regarding day and time, appointments during a day or assistance with making phone calls. Also, carers may be less anxious knowing that in unsafe situations, the CDN will provide warning signals to the persons with dementia. Measuring quality of life in carers is still not usual in psychosocial intervention studies in dementia (Moniz-Cook et al., 2008) and that is the reason that there is no specific dementia-related quality of life instrument for carers. Therefore, in this case a general health-related quality of life measure is suggested, for instance the Short-Form Health Survey scales (Ware and Sherbourne 1992), which have good psychometric properties. As an alternative one could also ask a single item on quality of life has been used, for instance: "All things taken together, how do you rate your overall quality of life?" People can be asked to give a grade for this or to answer on a five-point scale.

There exist many instruments measuring caregiver burden. An instrument that frequently has been used in carers of persons with dementia and that has good psychometric properties is the Sense of Competence Questionnaire (SCQ; Vernooij-Dassen 1993). There is also a short version (SSCQ; Vernooij-Dassen et al. 1999), consisting of seven items, that has shown sensitivity to change (van der Roest et al., 2008).

14.3.2.5 Measurement Instruments to Describe the Test Population

In the COGKNOW project we use several instruments to collect data on characteristics of the user-participants in the project. First, we use a self-composed questionnaire to inventory specific background characteristics (age, gender, living situation, education, etc.) and context characteristics (type of housing, neighbourhood, use of public transport, etc.). The Mini Mental State Examination (MMSE, Folstein et al., 1975; Roth et al., 1986) is used to assess the cognitive functioning of persons with dementia and the Global Deterioration Scale (GDS, Reisberg et al., 1982) to assess the severity of dementia. Both instruments are widely used and have good psychometric properties.

Furthermore, we used the Practitioners Assessment of Network Type (PANT) to identify the type of social support the person with dementia receives (Wenger and Tucker 2002). The use of services list was applied to assess the way people use formal services (frequency, type) and their satisfaction with it (Dröes 1996; Schulz 1991).

14.4 Experiences with the (Impact) Measures in the First Cycle of the Project

In the first cycle of the project 17 persons with dementia and carers participated (see for characteristics of participants Chapter 6). Persons with dementia and carers were interviewed separately by trained interviewers in their own homes. The complete interviews (background characteristics and questionnaires) took approximately one and a half hours to administer. This was also the maximum time we set to the interview duration, to not overburden persons with dementia and carers. In cases where more time was needed to complete the interview two sessions, on different days, were held.

All scheduled questionnaires for persons with dementia and carers were administered at all test sites, except for the Jalowiec Coping Scale for the person with dementia. This questionnaire, that consists of 60 items with statements on strategies to cope with a stressful situation, was considered too long for the persons with dementia. This questionnaire was used with carers without problems, though they also perceived it as quite tiring.

Many persons with dementia and carers posed questions regarding the necessity of administration of the many questionnaires. We therefore explicitly explained them the reason for collecting these data. In the first cycle we used the data to describe the characteristics and disabilities of the group of persons for whom the assistive technology is being developed. Some of the instruments were applied to test if they were appropriate to be included as impact measures at a later stage. In these cases we, for instance, tested if persons with dementia understood the questions. To help the persons with dementia to focus at the interview, we often used response cards. In our experience this made the questionnaires easier to administer in persons with dementia. The responses persons with dementia gave on the questionnaires showed satisfactory variation.

14.5 Conclusion

In the COGKNOW project, the final research cycle aims to evaluate the impact of the COGKNOW Day Navigator on autonomy and quality of life of persons with dementia. The evaluation study will take place at three test sites in three countries (the Netherlands, Northern Ireland and Sweden) with a total of 12 persons with dementia and their informal carers. Different research methods will be used to evaluate the impact: (standardized) questionnaires, semi-structured interviews, diaries and logging methods. In selecting standardized questionnaires, several notions were considered, such as what is the range of domains of life or functioning that are targeted with this device, what are characteristics of the target group (e.g. severity of dementia, are participants able to participate in an interview?) and are measuring instruments available for the intended impact, and if so, what are the psychometric properties of these instruments? Within the COGKNOW project we decided that for the main impact areas (autonomy and quality of life) we would use (standardized) questionnaires. Though the pilot we carried out with these instruments in the first cycle of the project was satisfying, we will have to stay alert to the total amount of questionnaires to be used in the final research cycle. We will have to find a balance between relevant questionnaires to answer the research questions on the one hand and the burden we put on persons with dementia and carers on the other hand.

Some of the questionnaires, the CANE and the Qol-AD, are administered in both persons with dementia and their carers. In this way, we are able to compare opinions from both perspectives. From previous studies we know that persons with mild dementia are very well able to indicate their needs, but it became clear that at some points they differ in their opinions from their carers (van der Roest et al., 2008). For example, people with dementia reported less needs than carers, and the agreement on objective needs areas (e.g. mobility, physical health) was better than on more subjective need areas (e.g. behaviour, alcohol abuse). In the semi-structured interviews we will therefore pay attention to both the persons with dementia and carers perspective for each area of support. In the interviews we will assess whether the CDN addresses the needs of persons with dementia in four areas, memory, social contact, activity and safety. By means of logging data we will assess the actual use of the CDN in daily life during the whole test period of 2 months.

A limitation of the impact measurement in the COGKNOW project is that it takes place during the development process of the assistive device. This means that the prototype tested will be restricted to the functions that are stable enough to be tested. Furthermore, there will be some practical restrictions (time available for testing, budget for acquiring test equipments and number of respondents in the test) that will make it impossible to conduct a large randomized controlled trial. However, as the aim of the COGKNOW project is to develop a cognitive prosthetic device together with potential end-users, iterative needs assessments, consultations between domain experts and system designers, and evaluations of different prototypes are very relevant for the development process. Once an end product of the assistive technology is available, it is recommended though to conduct a randomized controlled trial with a larger sample, to assess the general impact of the technology on the daily life of persons with dementia and carers. Since dementia is a progressive syndrome, it is to be expected that persons with dementia will deteriorate in one way or another during longer intervention periods. This is relevant for designing effect studies, because in this case also less deterioration in functioning than usual should be interpreted as a positive impact of the device. To prove the impact of the ICT device a control group is essential.

In selecting instruments to assess the impact of ICT interventions in dementia care, it is worthwhile to consult the European consensus on outcome measures for psychosocial interventions in dementia as recently published by the INTERDEM group (Moniz-Cook et al., 2008).

Appendix 1: Experienced Autonomy

I will now read to you a number of statements. I would like you to tell me whether you recognize these statements and to what degree they refer to your current situation.

The procedure is as follows. I will read each statement out aloud and tell you the answering categories. You are then asked to indicate with which answer you agree most. You can choose from the following five answer alternatives:

1. totally disagree
2. disagree
3. neither agree nor disagree
4. agree
5. totally agree

Instruction for Interviewer

Circle the answer for each statement given by the respondent.

		Totally disagree	Disagree	Neither agree nor disagree	Agree	Totally agree
1	I have little control over the things that happen to me[a]	1	2	3	4	5
2	There is really no way I can solve some of the problems I have[a]	1	2	3	4	5
3	There is little I can do to change many of the important things in my life[a]	1	2	3	4	5

		Totally disagree	Disagree	Neither agree nor disagree	Agree	Totally agree
4	I often feel helpless in dealing with the problems of life[a]	1	2	3	4	5
5	Sometimes I feel that I am being pushed around in life[a]	1	2	3	4	5
6	What happens to me in the future mostly depends on me[a]	1	2	3	4	5
7	I can do just about anything I really set my mind to do[a]	1	2	3	4	5
8	I feel I have difficulty performing everyday activities[b]	1	2	3	4	5
9	I am capable of deciding where I want to go[b]	1	2	3	4	5
10	I feel able to make decisions[b]	1	2	3	4	5
11	I feel capable of meeting my obligations[b]	1	2	3	4	5
12	I am sufficiently mobile to get where I want to go[b]	1	2	3	4	5

©Meiland and Dröes (2006).
[a]Pearlin and Schooler (1978)(Mastery Scale)
[b]Adjusted from WHOQOL100

Appendix 2: Dementia Coping Questionnaire

I am going to read to you a number of statements. I would like to know if you recognize these statements.

It works like this: I read each statement out aloud and I give you the possible answer categories. You then indicate which answer you most agree with. You can choose from the following four alternatives:

1. totally agree
2. somewhat agree
3. somewhat disagree
4. totally disagree

Instruction for Interviewer

Circle the number referring to the alternative mentioned by the respondent

		Totally agree	Somewhat agree	Somewhat disagree	Totally disagree
1	Since my memory problems were finally diagnosed, I have felt relieved	1	2	3	4
2	I do memory exercises (riddles and crossword puzzles)	1	2	3	4
3	I have a daily routine I stick to	1	2	3	4
4	I try to accomplish as much as I can on the days I feel well	1	2	3	4
5	I am getting older, so forgetfulness is normal	1	2	3	4
6	I generally try to think as little as possible about my problems	1	2	3	4
7	I avoid new situations and unfamiliar places	1	2	3	4
8	I withdraw from conversations; I am afraid I will forget what people have said	1	2	3	4
9	I am not ashamed of my illness and talk about it openly	1	2	3	4
10	I rely on others to remind me of appointments and obligations	1	2	3	4
11	I get scared when I think about my future	1	2	3	4
12	I try to laugh about my forgetfulness	1	2	3	4
13	I make lots of notes so I won't forget anything	1	2	3	4
14	My forgetfulness often annoys me	1	2	3	4
15	I am afraid of losing myself because of my memory problems	1	2	3	4
16	I know that my forgetfulness is an illness and it is not my fault	1	2	3	4
17	I have given up much social contact	1	2	3	4
18	My forgetfulness is embarrassing and I am ashamed of it	1	2	3	4
19	In case I don't know an answer, I respond with an appropriate saying	1	2	3	4
20	I try to make the best of my situation	1	2	3	4
21	When I think about my illness I become depressed or pessimistic	1	2	3	4
22	I discuss my fears and feelings with people I trust	1	2	3	4
23	I ignore my illness and the problems it causes	1	2	3	4
24	I have gathered as much information on my illness as possible	1	2	3	4

©Reinsersmann et al., VU Medical Center, Amsterdam, (2006)

References

ASTRID. (2000) ASTRID: A Guide to Using Technology within Dementia Care. Hawker publications, London.

Brod, M., Stewart, A., Sands, L., Walton, P. (1999) Conceptualisation and measurement of quality of life in dementia: The Dementia Quality of Life Instrument (DQOL). Gerontologist, 39: 25–35.

Dröes, R.M. (1996). Amsterdamse Ontmoetingscentra; een nieuwe vorm van ondersteuning voor dementerende mensen en hun verzorgers, Eindrapport 1996 [Amsterdam Meeting Centres: A new type of support for people with dementia and their carers, Final report 1996]. Thesis Publishers, Amsterdam.

Dröes, R.M., van Hout, H.P.J., van der Ploeg, E.S. (2004) Camberwell Assessment of Need for the Elderly (CANE). Revised Version (IV). Amsterdam: VU Free university medical hospital, Department of Psychiatry, EMGO institute.

Dröes, R.M., Meiland, F.J., Schmitz, M.J., van Tilburg, W. (March 2006) Effect of the Meeting Centres Support Program on informal carers of people with dementia: Results from a multicentre study. Aging and Mental Health, 10(2):112–124.

Dröes, R.M., Van Tilburg, W. (1998) Kwaliteit van zorg en kwaliteit van leven bij dementie. In: P. W. Huijbers, W. W. Van Santvoort (eds.) Conference Proceedings. Nederlands Instituut voor Gerontologie, The Netherlands, p. 28.102.

Ettema, T.P., Dröes, R.M., de Lange, J., Mellenbergh, G.J., Ribbe, M.W. (2005) A review of quality of life instruments used in dementia. Quality of Life Research, 14(3):675–686.

Folstein, M.F., Folstein, S.E., McHugh, P.R. (1975) "Mini-mental state". A practical method for grading the cognitive state of patients for the clinician. Journal of Psychiatric Research, 12: 189–198.

Health Council of the Netherlands. (2002) Dementie. Health Council of the Netherlands, The Hague.

Lauriks, S., Reinersmann, A., van der Roest, H.G. et al. (2007) Review of ICT-based services for identified unmet needs in people with dementia. Ageing Research Reviews, 6:223–246.

Lawton, M.P. (1991) A multidimensional view of quality of life in frail elders. In: J.E. Birren, J. Lubben, J.C. Rowe, D.E. Deutschmann (eds.) The Concept and Measurement of Quality of Life. Academic Press, New York, pp. 3–27.

Logsdon, R.G., Gibbons, L.E., McCurry, S.M., Teri, L. (1999) Quality of life in Alzheimer's disease: Patient and caregiver reports. Journal of Mental Health and Aging, 5(1):21–32.

Meiland, F.J.M., Dröes, R.M. (2006) Experienced Autonomy. VU Free University Medical Hospital, Department of Psychiatry, EMGO Institute, Amsterdam.

Miranda, C.I., Orrell, M. (2008) At Home with Dementia. European Association of Geriatric Psychiatry, Kos Island, Greece, p. 43.

Moniz-Cook, E., Vernooij-Dassen, M., Woods, R. et al (2008) A European consensus on outcome measures for psychosocial intervention research in dementia care. Aging and Mental Health, 12(10):14–29.

Nugent, C.D. (2007) ICT in the elderly and dementia. Editorial, Aging and Mental Health, 11(5):473–476.

Pearlin, L.I., Schooler, C. (1978) The structure of coping. Journal of Health and Social Behaviour, 19:2–21.

Rabins, P.V., Kasper, J.D. (1997) Measuring quality of life in dementia: Conceptual and practical issues. Alzheimer Disease and Associated Disorders, 11:100–104.

Reinersmann, A., Meiland, F.J.M., Dröes, R.M. (2006) Dementia Coping Questionnaire. VU Medical Center, Amsterdam.

Reisberg, B., Ferris, S., De Leon, M.J. et al (1982) The global deterioration scale for assessment of primary degenerative dementia. American Journal of Psychiatry, 139:1136–1139.

Reynolds, T., Thornicroft, G., Abas, M. et al (2000) Camberwell Assessment of Need for the Elderly (CANE): Development, validity and reliability. British Journal of Psychiatry, 176: 444–452.

Roth, M., Tym, E., Mountjoy, C.Q. et al. (1986) CAMDEX. A standardised instrument for the diagnosis of mental disorder in the elderly with special reference to the early detection of dementia. British Journal of Psychiatry, 149:698–709.

Schultz, C. (1991) Dementie onderzoek; een verkennende studie naar de verzorgers van dementerende bejaarden in Amsterdam. [Dementia research; an exploratory study among the carers of elderly people with dementia in Amsterdam.] PCA/Valeriuskliniek, Amsterdam, Unpublished Report.

Schölzel-Dorenbos, C.J.M., Ettema, T.P., Boelens-van der Knoop, E.C.C., Bos, J., Gerritsen, D.L., Hoogeveen, F., de Lange, J., Meihuizen, L., Dröes, R.M. (2007) Evaluating the outcome of psychosocial and farmacological interventions on quality of life of people with dementia: when to use what QoL instrument? International Journal of Geriatric Psychiatry, 22:511–519.

Shankar, K.K., Walter, M., Frost, D., Orrell, M.W. (1999) The development of a valid and reliable scale for rating anxiety in dementia (RAID). Aging and Mental Health, 3:39–49.

Spector, A., Thormgrimsen, L., Woods, B., Royan, L., Davies, S. et al (2003) A randomised controlled trial investigating the effectiveness of an evidence-based cognitive stimulation therapy programme for people with dementia. British Journal of Psychiatry, 183:356–54.

Teunisse, S., Derix, M.M. (1991) Measurement of activities of daily living in patients with dementia living at home: development of a questionnaire. Tijdschrift voor Gerontologie en Geriatrie [in Dutch], 22:201–203.

Van der Roest, H.G., Meiland, F.J.M., Maroccini, R., et al. (2007) Subjective needs of people with dementia: a review of the literature. International Psychogeriatrics 19:559–592.

Van der Roest, H.G., Meiland, F.J.M., van der Hout, H.P., Jonker, C., Dröes, R.M. (2008) Validity and reliability of the Dutch version of the Camberwell Assessment of Need for the Elderly in community-dwelling people with dementia. International Psychogeriatrics 20(6):1273–1290.

Vernooij-Dassen, M. (1993). Dementie en thuiszorg. Swets & Zeitlinger, Amsterdam/Lisse.

Vernooij-Dassen, M.J., Felling, A.J., Brummelkamp, E., Dauzenberg, M.G., van den Bos, G.A., Grol, R. (1999) Assessment of caregiver's competence in dealing with the burden of caregiving for a dementia patient: a Short Sense of Competence Questionnaire (SSCQ) suitable for clinical practice. Journal of the American Geriatrics Society, 47:256–257.

WHO SRPB Quality of Life Group (2002) WHOQOL-SRPB Field Test Instrument. Department of Mental Health and Substance Dependence, WHO, Geneva, Switzerland.

Ware, J.E., Sherbourne, C.D. (1992) The MOS 36-itme Short-Form Health Survey (SF-36): Conceptual framework and item selection. Medical Care, 30:473–483.

Wenger, G.C., Tucker, I. (2002) Using network variation in practice: identification of support network type. Health and Social Care in the Community, 10:28–35.

Chapter 15
Technology and Dementia: The Way Ahead

Jeffrey Kaye

You can never plan the future by the past
Edmund Burke [Irish statesman and philosopher (1729–1797)]
The future aint't what it used to be
Yogi Berra [US baseball player, coach, & manager (1925–)]

Abstract This chapter is an overview of the future state of the art in using technology to help people remain functionally independent and in their residence of choice. This is perceived to be the direction and ultimate goal of dementia treatment and prevention. Of course methods and new approaches gained in striving toward an era of prevention may be immediately applicable to those who unfortunately nevertheless may succumb to dementing illnesses as well. This chapter describes first what current and then prospective generations of senior's experiences and interactions can tell us about how technologies may be shaped and used in the future. This is followed by a vision of the future based on the view that the multiple technologies now available will continually undergo mixing and hybridization such that increasingly the home will become the basic unit of assessment and care provision in an environment of multifunctional ambient technology monitoring and health maintenance. Finally, key challenges to achieving this environment are described at the person level as well as the technical and systems level. Ultimately, these are perceived as challenges that can be surmounted ushering in an era of personalized health maintenance and care that also provides better population-based policy and management.

J. Kaye (✉)
Departments of Neurology and Biomedical Engineering, Oregon Center for Aging and Technology, Oregon Health and Science University, Portland, OR, USA
e-mail: kaye@ohsu.edu

M.D. Mulvenna, C.D. Nugent (eds.), *Supporting People with Dementia Using Pervasive Health Technologies*, Advanced Information and Knowledge Processing, DOI 10.1007/978-1-84882-551-2_15, © Springer-Verlag London Limited 2010

15.1 Introduction

This chapter is about predicting the future – how to take the vectors of change among an aging population and visualize their destinations based on technological innovation and adaptation. On the one hand, it is easy to speculate and discuss what the future may bring and how we might get there – you can't prove a prognosticator wrong until their future vision actually arrives or fails to materialize. At the same time, it is extraordinarily difficult to predict with precision what the future holds as it is not only the technologies that evolve rapidly, but more importantly the culture and practices surrounding these technologies that ultimately determine their uptake. As a starting point, clearly the chapters in this book have presented a wide range of current and near term developments in the fields of geriatrics, cognitive impairment, and the use of technology for assessing and intervening among the attendant chronic conditions associated with brain aging. These form the context for considering directions for the future. In this chapter, we will focus primarily on seniors who are *not* impaired or only mildly impaired and living independently as these are the individuals most at risk, most likely to be living with an impaired spouse or helping relatives or friends in the community and hopefully, provided with a wide array of tools to not only mitigate existing cognitive impairment but also prevent their own cognitive decline.

15.2 What Current Seniors Tell Us About the Future

In considering what the future may hold for the role of technology in dementia care, one of the most important aspects to consider is not just the technology per se, but the factors that play a role in the *adoption and dissemination* of new technologies. There are many factors that can play a role in this uptake including education, familiarity, and experience with prior related technologies, perception of usefulness, cognitive and physical abilities, and cost.

In considering the use of technology by current seniors an important starting point is to examine what devices or technologies have been widely used, as well as those that have not found wide uptake. In particular, much attention has been paid to the rising, but still low frequency of computer usage among those over age 65. This is a worldwide trend. For example, it is estimated that approximately 56% of people aged 64–72 go online in the USA (Pew Internet Survey 2009). In Europe, the number is lower overall. Among the EU27, 29% of those aged 65–74 undertake any Internet-related activities, but the range of online users is quite variable across European Union countries (Ala-Mutka et al. 2008). In this context, beyond computer and Internet use there are few systematic surveys of current seniors and the devices or technologies that they use. A recent US study surveying the use of common household devices (including computers) found among the oldest old that televisions, microwave ovens, and answering machines were the most commonly used with 97, 80, and 57% being frequent users of these devices, respectively (Calvert et al. 2009). On the other hand, cell phones and computers were only used frequently by 13 and 18%, respectively. Importantly, of those that didn't have personal computers, 84% did not wish to acquire one. The reasons for this were not explicitly studied in this report. However, other work has suggested that cognitive abilities, computer self-efficacy, and computer anxiety are important mediators of computer use among the aging (Czaja et al. 2006).

One of the most striking contexts that cuts across most of this work is the fact that the current generation of seniors currently live in a world that contains many technologies that have only emerged during the last decades of their lives. Many of these are key to the many approaches taken toward assessment and management of dementia. Most of them are not familiar to this demographic. Consider that the current 80-year-olds were born in 1929 and spent their most active years of formal education up until about 1960. Further interaction with evolving technologies of course continued to occur in the community and in the workplace; although in this generation fewer women were engaged in the professional or technical workforce. This generation formally entered "old age" by virtue of being over age 65 in the mid-1990s. This period for the current octogenarian generation is precisely the time when such current take-it-for-granted capabilities afforded by technologies such as personal computers, digital media (photos, video, music, etc.), and the Internet only emerged on a wide scale and importantly on a commercially successful basis. An important point here is that the aging-associated experience of seniors is key.

Obviously, this does not mean that all seniors are technophobes or are incapable or unwilling to learn to use new devices or integrate them into their routines. An American Association for Retired Persons survey confirms this specifically for ambient monitoring, for example, showing that among seniors over age 65 (a younger "old" demographic), 56% of respondents said they would be willing to use an "electronic device that lets someone who lives outside your home know if you are okay, or if your daily routine changes" (AARP Healthy@Home 2008). In addition, there are many examples of seniors learning to use computers, Skype their grandchildren, and participate in online communities. However, one must also keep in mind the steep curve of cognitive change after age 65 leading potentially to as many as 50% of those aged 85 and older to experience mild cognitive impairment. It is thus likely that for these individuals and younger elderly with earlier onset of cognitive decline, even if motivated, unless the technology strongly relies on past patterns and experience, the use of new technology or devices will be less successfully adopted and ultimately useful. On the other hand, when legacy technologies are integrated with new approaches one may not only successfully adopt new paradigms but also gain immensely from this use.

One instructive example comes from a study of medication adherence where the technology chosen was the familiar multi-compartment pillbox. This simple common reminding device was instrumented so that when the doors of the compartments were opened an electronic switch was triggered allowing for time-stamping of the event. The data was sent wirelessly through a Bluetooth radio contained in the bottom of the box (with the rest of the electronics). Thus, the recording and reporting of medication taking could be facilitated as well as the provision of potential feedback about performance since the device was similar to what was already in use, portable and could operate in near real time (Hayes et al. 2006). Using this device the authors found that among a group of cognitively intact, independently living seniors, those who fell into the lower end of the cognitively normal spectrum had significantly worse medication adherence (Hayes et al. 2009). The importance of this for our present review is that using a more complex or new device, it would be more difficult to differentiate whether their failure was the result of cognitive dysfunction itself or the inability to use the device or both. The importance of these examples is not that technology cannot be helpful. In fact it was highly informative in this case. The key implication is that in order for technologies to be used effectively they need to be formulated such that they are generation appropriate from a practical standpoint. From this point of view the current generation of seniors is not likely in large numbers by themselves to successfully adopt new technologies. Thus, for current seniors in the next 5–10 years, it may be that the repurposing or reconfiguration of familiar legacy devices or modifying only subtly longer standing practices may be more successful than invention of new ways of doing things.

15.3 What Future Seniors Tell Us About the Future

As noted in the preceding section, practically speaking, much of the current technology available to use may need to be packaged in a retrospective way for successful adoption by current seniors except in special cases such as for retired engineers, early adopters, or those with lifelong patterns of cognitive flexibility. Of course their children, the Baby Boomers, and their grand children, Generation X, who are involved in their care (and their own care as they age) can and will use existing and rapidly evolving technology as well. Accordingly, the future benefit of technology in the coming decade and beyond for dementia will accrue more to these next generations of seniors, especially the Baby Boomers, than the current older generation. This generation has also been called the "Sandwich Generation" referring to being squeezed between caring for parents and tending to their growing children while maintaining a job and personal life for themselves. Their experience with technology is also wedged between that of their parents having seen, for example, both the advent of TV, instant photography, the microwave oven, and the cardiac pacemaker and the technologies that most defined their children's early experience such as cellular phones, personal computers, videogames, text messaging, and the expanded use of the Internet. Thus, the framework for the future adoption and use of technology by future generations of seniors and their carers must be placed in this context. Importantly here, one must consider that some technologies are very slow to expand while others become rapidly incorporated into society and everyday use. The pace of these transitions is the result of many forces ranging from pure practical utility to politics and economics. In any event, ongoing review of this background and context is key to gauging over time the likelihood of realizing any vision of the future.

15.4 An Idealized Future

Appropriately, a review of topics with regard to technology and dementia is often distributed (as in this book) into aspects related to assessment and then interventions. They are often further divided specifically into sub-domains of assessment relative to cognition and function and interventions related to alerting and safety, medical, and social support. Other overarching topics such as ethics and economics are also needed to round out the review. In this projection of the future one could map onto this outline anticipated developments in each specific area such as the future development of alerting devices or social networking interventions. Doing so would reflect the current piecemeal and disconnected state of independent aging aids and technologies. However, another way to consider what will occur in the future is how all of the existing and promising threads of technology will come together. This trend is likely because in general this has been the evolution of many technologies and as suggested above, it is when technologies are woven into the existing stream of daily activity that they are most readily effective, quickly adopted, and widely disseminated.

With this perspective in mind, I propose that the future will see a convergence of technologies in several domains that ultimately will be considered a routine part of the home environment and health maintenance. These technology systems form the basis for aware or context-sensitive assessment and prompting in the stream of everyday life. Popular terms for this concept are "pervasive" or "ubiquitous computing technologies" or "ambient technology." Much of this technology environment conceptually comes from the tradition of the "smart home." The term "smart home" has been used most often to describe the general concept of a home that is outfitted with technology that automates the detection of events and performs activities or functions for the person living in that structure without them having to consciously act. In the building industry this home automation (sometimes called "domotics") is most commonly focused on environmental engineering (e.g., cooling/heating, lighting, home entertainment systems, alarms). In the health care sphere the concept is generally enlarged and used to describe a home where technology is placed or used to automate capture of data or provide interventions relevant to health. This ranges from automated assessment of motion to detect relevant events such as walking, falls, or general activity levels (e.g., using passive IR sensors around the home), activities of daily living such as medication taking (e.g., instrumentation of a pillbox or dispenser), physiological data such as vital signs (e.g., monitoring via an embedded scale in the floor or a bed mat), or degree of socialization (e.g., using motion sensors measuring amount of time out of home, or with phone monitoring, number of relevant phone calls). The system seamlessly connects to other devices such as home appliances, cell phones, or medical devices that may change over time or intermittently leave the home. Ideally these technologies talk to one another and form an intelligent sensor net that acts in the background to unobtrusively identify ongoing patterns of health or intermittent acute events. Data from this system is either fed back to the person directly or sent to a professional or family member for further evaluation and action. The outcomes of any actions or interventions are in turn automatically reviewable and appropriately modified, immediately or in near real time. Most importantly, because of the continuous and personalized nature of the data derived from this kind of system, trends over time can be discerned with much greater precision allowing for the realization of true proactive or preventive medicine.

This setup not only is multifunctional in terms of the domains and functions that can be assessed and acted upon but also provides the opportunity to transition its degree and levels of support through the aging process, from independent living to more assisted levels of need. At the level of organizations and society the ready availability of real-time data from thousands of households provides the opportunity to plan and deliver more effectively health programs for the community at large.

15.5 The Future Is Almost Now

The seeds of this future in the dementia care world are present in several current developments. Perhaps, the fullest instantiation of this direction is found in the evolution of the use of technology in assisted care and nursing facilities. Aside from the obvious alarm pull cord in a bathroom or sensor-tripped exit door locks, there are now several companies marketing full end-to-end multifunctional "smart" systems for monitoring residents and staff and integrating this data into the operation of the facility. The first such approach and among the most complete was established within an assisted living facility in 2000 by Elite Care in Milwaukee, Oregon (Elite Care 2009). The residence, Oatfield Estates, is a congregate housing-assisted living facility in which each resident and staff member wears an infrared/radiofrequency badge; beds are outfitted with load cells. The data from this sensor net is used for location monitoring, tracking weight and time in bed, alerting functions, as well as maintaining the operations of the facility. The data is all electronically presented to the staff whose own activity is assessed and can be reviewed by management. The management, for example, has a policy that when each staff member engages a resident, they typically need to spend more than a few seconds with the person. The time of resident–staff interaction can be automatically charted to gauge adherence to this policy using this system. The environment is also monitored relative to a resident's location including temperature, utility usage, and movement about the grounds of the estate. If a resident is in the communal kitchen and has been identified to be a cooking risk, the system will alert a staff member that they need to check on what's happening in the kitchen; otherwise they can continue unsupervised with their work. If a resident wanders to the perimeter this may set off a sprinkler system in their path as a means of keeping the resident from wandering away (and thus alleviating the need to have locks on all the doors). Importantly, the daily data from the system is also available not only to the staff but also with permission from the resident for the family through an online family portal.

This existing model in various versions has been implemented at least partially in other assisted care settings (and expanded by Elite Care). This institutionally based trend has begun to be expanded to individual homes providing the opportunity for a senior or family member to directly design and engage a home-based care management system on their own. The roots of this trend started in initial community pilot programs developed only in the last 10 years. For example, the "Opening Doors for Seniors" project in the West Lothian District of Scotland (Bowes and McColgan 2006) demonstrated how selected alerting and safety systems (e.g., call alarms, temperature sensors, motion sensors) could be installed in home and coupled with telemedicine and local care managers providing increased sense of well-being as well as cost savings primarily through delaying more expensive institutional types of care and acute medical encounters. There are now several thousand West Lothian residents using versions of this system. This and other similar projects have generally focused on those identified to have already some risk for imminent failure and a move to institutional care. This triage of use is appropriately driven by the economic realities of the cost of installing and maintaining systems as well as the yet to be proven benefit of preventive monitoring in those who are only at risk because of age, but are otherwise still quite functional. However, in the future one can envision not only applying these technologies to the homes of high-risk seniors but also having the systems as a part of almost all residences.

There are few examples where ambient in-home monitoring of the residences of independent seniors *without* focused health problems (dementia, diabetes, heart disease, etc.) or at high safety risk have been deployed beyond a few demonstration homes. However, one effort that has achieved this goal at least in several hundred active independent seniors has been reported in a project in Portland, Oregon (Kaye et al. 2008). In this Technology and Aging project the Oregon Center for Aging & Technology (ORCATECH) created a simple home-based platform of infrared motion sensors and contact sensors placed strategically about the homes of seniors living independently in the community (most often in retirement apartments). Importantly these seniors were computer literate, i.e., could reliably send and receive email, and if not, they were taught to be capable of effectively using a home computer. This provided access to being able to communicate on a regular basis (generally weekly) via email about health-related functions such as falls, mood changes, or medication adjustments. It also provided a means for unobtrusively assessing fine motor function such as mouse movements or keyboard strokes as well as higher order cognitive functions such as a person's typical performance upon repeatedly playing online games or other activities. The system's data is sent wirelessly from the home via broadband connections to a central research server for analysis. Special custom software remotely manages the project allowing the monitoring team to "see" into the home and determine the status of a system in real time (e.g., battery life, sensor firing history). This ubiquitous in-home platform has been running in the community for over 2 years as of this writing. This project suggests both the power and the limitations of this model for the future. First, much of the data coming from these homes is acquired without direct query of the residents – it is truly ambient. Thus, a wide range of daily activity patterns such as total activity in a day, time in bed, time in the bathroom, number of outings, and walking speed are acquired which have known health implications. For example, total activity and speed of walking acquired over several months with this system have been shown to differentiate seniors with mild cognitive impairment compared to those that remain cognitively intact (Hayes et al. 2008). Second, the frequency and fine granularity of the data provides an opportunity to evaluate true within-person change in real time. This unique character of the data provides the opportunity to not only examine gross mean differences at single points in time but uniquely allows analysis of time trends and time variant variability. By its nature the number of captured instances of events is very large allowing much greater power in analysis. For example, typical clinical studies of walking speed obtain a single measure per year. In the current paradigm, thousands of walking episodes per person per year may be obtained. Third, new ways of looking at problems can be afforded. For example, falls, a highly feared event for healthy seniors, as well as an increased risk for dementia patients are largely unpredictable. With this kind of system, one can not only better pinpoint a fall, but search for activity and other kinds of data from minutes to months before the event for clues about precedent circumstances leading to the fall. Despite this potential, there are considerable challenges to realizing a more widespread generalized application of ambient computing in the homes of seniors.

15.6 Realizing a Future of Ambient Home Technology for Seniors – Person-Centered Considerations

As one moves from the organized institutional community to the free-standing household in the wider community setting issues of scalability currently hinder the full build-out of this kind of technology for wider adoption. There are several barriers that will need to be overcome, but several trends and possible solutions may enable the full potential of this flexible real-world model to become widely adopted. In the remaining sections of this chapter these major trends and forces will be highlighted.

One of the first framing issues that is faced in building out ambient home health technology to the wider community is the increasing heterogeneity of the population that can use and benefit from these services. These population features include (1) personal factors such as a person's level of education, familiarity with technology, comfort with new devices, and economic status; (2) health status such as cognitive function, chronic conditions, mobility, and sensory abilities (hearing and vision); and (3) physical residence or environmental factors such as whether a person lives in a remote rural area or a high-rise apartment block. These considerations naturally lead to several major technical challenges that through anticipated research and development could greatly facilitate change.

First, one of the major considerations with regard to future seniors and their unique characteristics is what their legacy of education and experience with technologies has been. Although there is evidence that the next generation of seniors – the Baby Boomers – may be more technically sophisticated and thus more able to take advantage of new technologies than current seniors, one must keep in mind that new technological developments will continue to evolve, and thus the same lack of widespread adoption of home computers and Internet use that characterizes current seniors may be replaced by a new lack of uptake among the next generation of seniors by new technologies that as we read this we have yet to envision. One already sees this to some extent in the social networking sphere where, for example, 55–64-year-olds make up 12% of Facebook Internet domain search traffic while those age 65 or older make up only 3% (Ignite Social Media 2009). One currently will commonly hear those over 50 wondering "how would anyone have the time to Twitter all day?" The ability of future seniors to adopt new technology or ways of living is difficult to predict. Some technologies have enduring legacies and once basically learned allow an individual to continue to adapt as the technology evolves. Thus, a current senior that learned to drive a car in the 1940s, if not demented can still drive a contemporary car. Importantly and instructive for predicting the future, the new technology in the car is largely invisible to the senior of today and in fact generally improves the driving experience. Thus, personal computers, cell phones, and digital cameras may function in this way such that the current "smart phone" or personal digital assistant, if considered as a mash-up of these several platforms (now containing all these functions), can be readily adopted even by a Baby Boomer because the underlying functions of the individual devices have been a part of their lives for some time already.

In addition to the basic familiarity and comfort level with using a system it is clear that this system needs to adapt to the variety of generally accruing and unfortunately increasing number of common chronic conditions experienced with typical aging. Thus, one of the basic barriers to much of senior technology adoption tracks along two interacting lines. First, the person's cognitive ability to multitask and receive novel information for immediate action does not improve with time. This is particularly the case for common aging-associated declines in working memory and executive function that are important to effective learning and operation of new devices or technologies. Second, the person's basic ability to physically act is subject to changes in energy level, circadian rhythms, and pure physical ability. Any new systems or technology needs to allow for these aging health and physical factors.

Finally, there is a wide range of environments that older people inhabit. The isolated senior that lives in a rural area although potentially being able to benefit greatly from technology by bringing the outside world to their home also exemplifies the challenge of setting up ambient technologies in their home since at a minimum in this scenario one needs to service a potentially widely dispersed area. More than one truck-roll per residence to setup and service homes across wide geographic areas currently is not a viable business model. Thus, new technologies will need to be simple to set up, operable without much if any training, and very reliable. Similarly, the urban setting also creates challenges simply related to physical or environmental circumstances. The same setup and maintenance issues in more rural settings also apply to this environment. In addition, urban specific issues are also present. For example, current wireless technologies which may be key to future build-out of large networks of homes may not provide reliable service to all those located in the "canyons" of large apartment blocks. This last example brings us to consider the interface of the characteristics of the senior and the technologies and opportunities that the society in which that person lives that are available to realize a new technology-assisted independent living future.

15.7 Realizing a Future of Ambient Home Technology for Seniors – Technology and System Transformations

Evident from the discussion above is the fact that there are promising threads of development that suggest a fully integrated home platform may be achievable in the near future. The current low penetration of contemporary technology use at least with regard to some aspects of ICT will likely increase dramatically among the next generation of seniors and their carers. As the aging demographic continues to shift increasing attention is being paid to the needs of an aging population. However, some of the most basic key challenges to scalability of the multifunctional ambient technology monitoring and health maintenance model are technical and cut across a wide range of capabilities in realizing the assessment and intervention environment of the future. They are anticipated to be solved in part because they are a part of general trends in technology or health care, and as noted above, they are already available to some extent in institutional settings or community-wide experiments or demonstration sites. In addition, across multiple domains there are active developments in building out standards that will be needed to achieve interoperability whether in device communication protocols or electronic record keeping. Finally, with more efficient and accurate technology along with standards will come the ability to compare evidence on a level playing field which can then be used to drive markets and government decisions based on what truly works. This will ultimately fuel wide adoption and dissemination.

In this final section I outline six areas that will need to significantly change to realize a seamless ambient health maintenance system scaled to any community of seniors (or adults in general). Fortunately, most of these areas are in fact already trending toward needed change. One of the first issues will be the need for improved communication infrastructure, specifically broadband access (e.g., DSL, cable, WiMAX, satellite). This is crucial because for real-time data analysis and interventions based on these analyses, as well as timely sharing of data by multiple stakeholders fast, reliable, high bandwidth connectively at a reasonable price will be required. Currently, there is a wide variation not only by country but within a country as well. In addition, there are wide differences in speed and cost per bit. As an example, compare broadband capabilities in Japan and Switzerland (Correa 2007). In 2007 broadband penetration in Switzerland had reached 68 subscribers per 100 people (among the highest rates in Europe). Japan had 52 broadband subscribers per 100 people. One might conclude that broadband in Switzerland was more advanced. However, although a smaller proportion subscribe to broadband in Japan, its residents have access to a much more robust at less cost network. Thus, in Japan 100 mbps fiber optic service is available to 75% of residents, typically for about $27/month (USD), while the fastest connection widely available in Switzerland was 2.4 mbps DSL service at a price of approximately $52/month. This field's capabilities are rapidly evolving. Although the rate of proliferation of coverage at greater speeds and reduced cost will be variable, the general direction will be that increasingly more users will be covered while costs per bit decrease.

The second major needed change of importance is a general improvement in the many home-based sensor technologies available. One of the major considerations in successful continuous monitoring is whether assessments can be performed inadvertently and unobtrusively as part of the stream of everyday activities of living or more minimally obtrusive sensors or devices need to be engaged. Often, this is perceived of as a dichotomy between wearable (body-worn) versus environmental sensors. As sensors become smaller, cheaper, with lower power requirements, and with multifunction capabilities including the ability to be self-organizing, and maintaining, the practical distinction among different sensor types relative to user interaction becomes blurred. Thus, a small sensor if very cheap can be embedded in the environment as well as worn in multiple locations in different form factors. Being inexpensive makes loss of a device less of a tragedy and supports the virtues of redundancy. If sensors are self-organizing they can gauge their function relative to other sensors in the environment as they change or even malfunction. This trend in technical capabilities is particularly important moving forward for a particular problem that needs to be practically solved in community-based monitoring. This is the "multiperson" problem. Thus, when there is more than one person in a household one needs a reliable means for differentiating which actions belong to a particular person. This assumes that direct video visualization would not be widely used (although in some instances anonymised, "deformed" imaging may be allowed). Development in this technology domain is difficult to predict. Since most devices are still often conceived of as being directed toward specific problems such as fall detection or pill reminding, the underlying development concept of how these technologies should be further designed to interact as a unified network has not been the rule.

A third major barrier to the development of more interactive sensor and activator technology systems is being overcome due to positive developments in recent years toward the development of technical standards. This effort has been led by a number of groups and organizations such as the International Telecommunications Union (International Telecommunications Union 2009), the Wireless Sensor Working Group, IEEE, TC9 Technical Committee on Sensor Technology, Instrumentation and Measurement Society (Wireless Sensor Working Group 2009), the Continua Alliance (Continua 2009), the IHE Initiative (Integrating the Healthcare Enterprise 2009), and HL7 (Health Level 7 2009). Embedded in the need for technical standards is the question of how much open source development will occur. When systems become proprietary, in general this stifles rapid growth and spin-offs as time is spent developing "around" these bottlenecks and new cycles of development need to be played out.

Along with technical standards for devices are standards for the data that may come from these systems. In this regard, a fourth trend is the growth in electronic medical record capabilities. In general there appear to be two trends that will converge and be necessary for further growth of multifunctional ambient technology monitoring and health maintenance. First, the more formal health institutions have traditionally owned or managed individual health records. These have been increasingly transitioned from paper into electronic medical record (EMR) systems for use by the medical establishment during health care transactions. At the same time, on the home-front, individuals may increasingly archive their own information into systems ranging from personal profiles (e.g., Facebook, MySpace) to financial records and music libraries. A trend in line with this personal archiving is the development of personal health records (PHR). Many companies are developing and offering this service such as Google Health, Microsoft Health Vault, or Indivo – Dossia. If true interoperability and controlled sharing across these various record systems and the platforms used to maintain them is achieved there will be a blurring between the formal EMR and the PHR. The creation and routine population of these record systems with large amounts of data that may be derived from ambient health systems further sets up the potential to provide massive amounts of data not only at the individual level but at the population and health and welfare systems level as well.

In order to optimally analyze and use the data derived from home systems an increasing need will be a fifth trend – increasing facility with data storage, retrieval, meaningful analysis, and presentation to end users. Within each of these areas are several sub-domains of development such as network management, data security, data visualization, and statistical inference methodology. In the context of this chapter one critical area to highlight is the domain of data fusion. Simply stated, how does one best fuse the multiple constantly changing data streams from many sensors working contemporaneously as well as legacy data from previous days, weeks, or even years? In addition, ideally one also wants to call upon larger metadata from population-based experience. Initially, most of these data handling challenges will be handled with simple solutions. Data streams will be multiple, but may still use restricted channels such as simple combinations of motion activity and physiologic data across coarse-grained time epochs (days or weeks). Increasingly along with computing power and knowledge of optimized efficient algorithms, over time greater sophistication will be gained in specifying events and trends. Inclusion of data referring to other significant people in the person's life and social sphere can then expand the paradigm of health care to include not only the individual but also the dyads and other units of personal interaction. Obviously, these massive amounts of data will require in parallel growing new networks to manage and distribute this information.

These fundamental trends in data handling and extraction lead us to the final challenging trend and need that naturally derives from the maturing of home-based ambient assessment and management technologies. This is the need to infuse the entire clinical research enterprise with these kinds of technologies. This is critical in order to create the evidence base for what is effective or not. It includes improving clinical trial conduct as well as striving for real-time event captured epidemiology (Kaye 2008). Accordingly, clinical research methodology must fundamentally incorporate these new methods. We need to see the typical clinical study no longer being for example a brief cognitive test on a single brief visit to a clinic or even the home followed by months of waiting for events to occur that are then self reported following an intervention that we often cannot verify as to whether the treatment has been followed faithfully. What is more we need to see this clinical research model propagated on a large population-based scale. The degree to which this is achieved will translate into the ready interpretation of data that is immediately relevant to the person in their natural community environment in real time. This then enables the realization of true personalized medicine. Thus contrary to some who may be concerned that technology infused health care leads to depersonalization, multifunctional ambient monitoring, and health maintenance technology provides the opportunity to create over a lifetime a large personal database that pertains to the individual specifically. Expert decision support can then be based on knowledge of all prior events and trends not only derived from population averages (which would also be readily available) but also from individual level data from the person at home. On the larger, societal scale there are also benefits to be gained in that one can also plan more appropriately for public health purposes based on data-driven individual events at the household level. This creates the capability to span the ecosystem of health care management from the micro-climate of an individual's personal cloud to a population's moving front.

Acknowledgments The author's work was supported by grants from the U.S. National Institute on Aging (Grants: R01AG024059, P30 AG024978, and P30AG008017), The Department of Veterans Affairs, and Intel Corporation.

References

AARP. (2009) Healthy@Home; http://assets.aarp.org/rgcenter/il/healthy_home.pdf, accessed July 14, 2009.

Ala-Mutka, K., Punie, Y., Redecker, C. (2008) Digital Competence for Lifelong Learning, Policy Brief. Office for Official Publications of the European Communities, Luxembourg.

Bowes, A., McColgan, G. (2006) Smart Technology and Community Care for Older People: Innovation in West Lothian, Scotland. Scotland, Age Concern Scotland, Edinburgh.

Calvert, J.F., Kaye, J., Leahy, H.K., Carlson, N. (2009) Technology use by rural and urban oldest old. Technology and Health Care, 17:1–11.

Continua Health Alliance. (2009) http://www.continuaalliance.org/, accessed, July 30, 2009.

Correa, D.K. (2007) Assessing Broadband in America: OECD and ITIF Broadband Rankings. Information and Technology and Innovation Foundation. http://www.itif.org/files/BroadbandRankings.pdf, accessed, July 1, 2009.

Czaja, S.J., Charness, N., Fisk, A.D., Hertzog, C., Nair, S.N., Rogers, W.A., Sharit, J. (2006) Factors predicting the use of technology: Findings from the Center for Research and Education on Aging and Technology Enhancement (CREATE). Psychology and Aging, 21(2):333–352.

Elite Care. (2009) http://www.elitecare.com/, accessed, July 17, 2009.

Hayes, T.L., Hunt, J.M., Adami, A., Kaye, J.A. (2006) An electronic pillbox for continuous monitoring of medication adherence. Conference Proceedings: Engineering in Medicine and Biology Society, 1:6400–6403.

Hayes, T., Abendroth, F., Adami, A., Pavel, M., Zitzelberger, T., Kaye, J. (2008) Unobtrusive assessment of activity patterns associated with mild cognitive impairment. Alzheimer's & Dementia, 4(6):395–405.

Hayes, T.L., Larimer, N., Adami, A., Kaye, J.A. (2009) Medication Adherence in Healthy Elders: Small Cognitive Changes Make a Big Difference. Journal of Aging & Health, In Press.

Health Level 7 (HL7). (2009) http://www.hl7.org, accessed, July 30, 2009.

Ignite Social Media. (2009) http://s3.amazonaws.com/ignitesma/ignitewebsite/2009-social-network-analysis-report.pdf, accessed, August 2, 2009.

Integrating the Healthcare Enterprise (IHE). (2009) http://www.ihe.net, accessed, July 30, 2009.

International Telecommunications Union. (2009) ISO/IEEE 11073 Standards for Medical Device Communication. http://www.itu.int/itudoc/itu-t/workshop/e-health/addinfo/info009.html, Accessed, July 30, 2009.

Kaye, J., Hayes, T., Zitzelberger, T., Yeargers, J., Pavel, M., Jimison, H., Larimer, N., Payne-Murphy, J., Earl, E., Wild, K., Boise, L., Williams, D., Lundell, J., Dishman, E. (2008) Deploying wide-scale in-home assessment technology. In: A. Mihailidis, J. Boger, H. Kautz, L. Normie (eds.) Technology and Aging: Selected Papers from the 2007 International Conference on Technology and Aging. IOS Press, Amsterdam, The Netherlands, pp. 19–26.

Kaye, J. (2008) Home-based technologies: A new paradigm for conducting dementia prevention trials. Alzheimer's & Dementia, 4:p. S60–S66.

Wireless Sensor Working Group. (2009) IEEE, TC9 Technical Committee on Sensor Technology, Instrumentation and Measurement Society. http://grouper.ieee.org/groups/1451/5/, accessed, July 30, 2009.

Index

M.D. Mulvenna, C.D. Nugent (eds.), *Supporting People with Dementia Using*
Pervasive Health Technologies, Advanced Information and Knowledge Processing,
DOI 10.1007/978-1-84882-551-2, © Springer-Verlag London Limited 2010

Lightning Source UK Ltd.
Milton Keynes UK
UKOW031850130313

207613UK00004B/97/P